Morgane Leten

Decode Your Cycle

Harness Your Natural Hormones and Thrive Through Every Menstrual Phase

Lannoo

Here's to strong women,
may we know them,
may we be them,
may we raise them.

AMY REES ANDERSON

For my daughter Lola and all girls and women who have the right to accurate knowledge to discover the power of their cycle.

When I wrote this book, I was pregnant with my daughter. Both the writing and my pregnancy lasted about nine months. I am very grateful that my daughter has given me the strength and energy to make this happen.

This book contains information about the menstrual cycle and female health. It is not medical advice. The (personal) tips and insights are only intended as support. The information in this book is also not intended as a tool for making a (self-)diagnosis. If you have any medical questions, complaints or symptoms, consult your treating physician, so that you can receive a professional examination, diagnosis and, if necessary, medical care.

This book discusses women and the menstrual cycle. However, not only women have a uterus, but also trans men and non-binary individuals can experience bleeding. In the book, we use female pronouns, but of course we don't want to exclude anyone.

CONTENT: DECODE YOUR CYCLE

Why this book?

THE BENEFITS OF LIVING ACCORDING TO YOUR CYCLE

If you learn to use your menstrual cycle like I have been doing in recent years, you will notice that your cycle works like a compass; it always points in the right direction. By knowing your cycle better, you gain more insight into who you are and what is important to you.

As women, we experience greater hormonal fluctuations and these affect how we feel and perform. Women don't have a daily cycle like men, but a monthly cycle. But our patriarchal society pays little attention to that. Many women are also unaware of how their hormonal cycle affects their energy levels and mood swings throughout the month. The cause of this ignorance isn't hard to find. For generations, we have had to hear that health complaints related to the menstrual cycle are inherent to being a woman. And that is why women have been suffering in silence for years.

And there's the rub, it doesn't have to be that way. Your menstrual health is an important indicator of your overall health. In other words: if you experience a lot of menstrual pain or if it lasts for a long time, there is definitely something wrong with your body. Five years ago, I didn't know that either, just like 75 percent of women who have little to no knowledge about this subject. So don't feel bad or ignorant if you didn't know this either. It's time to turn the tide. I have suffered a lot myself from complaints that affected my self-confidence and relationships. I am so grateful that I am now pregnant with a daughter and that I can pass on all this information to her. My hope is that she can make better decisions and understand all the options to determine what is best for her. By creating more awareness and sharing knowledge about the menstrual cycle, women will realize that they can also use their cycle to their advantage to strengthen their position in the world.

THIS BOOK

I don't believe in miracles, but I do believe in getting to know your body, mapping out your cycle (specifically your ovulation) and following a balanced lifestyle by living according to the four seasons of your cycle.

This is, in my opinion, a story about hope. Hope to truly get to know your own body, empower yourself with thorough information, and thus give yourself the tools to truly give your body what it needs. You deserve it, both.

So welcome to this journey of discovering your natural cycle, where you finally learn to empower yourself. After a chapter about the basics of the female body, I will take you through the four seasons and tell you about the many unknown benefits of each phase. How is your energy, mood and libido during each phase, and how can you respond to them? Yes, it is definitely possible! How can you best exercise according to your cycle and how does your cycle affect your sleep? Which hormones are in charge and what impact do they have? I'll also be talking about how to eat according to your cycle; you're definitely not the only one who is overwhelmed by intense hunger just before your period.

And of course, I'll discuss all possible health complaints that may arise and how to deal with them. In addition to my own experiences, I will share those of other women, such as Nicole Jardim, Trix Eden Breuls, Eva Daeleman, Hilde De Baerdemaeker, Nouchka De Maeyer, Natasha Casteleyn, Ellen Kegels, Lynn Van Royen and Kim Clijsters. The goal is for you to be able to map out your own cycle every month after reading this book.

You can then live more in tune with your own body, with the seasons of your cycle. It will make you a stronger and happier woman.

MY STORY

As women, why do we only get full medical attention once we decide to have children? Only then should we take folic acid, live healthily and drink less alcohol. But what about women who just want to feel good every day, regardless of pregnancy, and have pain-free periods each month?

It's a question that I ask myself more and more, so many years after getting my first period, and one that I often hear from other women as well. The day before my fifteenth birthday, I had my first period. I was so happy. Finally, I felt like I belonged. What I didn't know yet was that my period was not going to make life easy for me. I experienced heavy bleeding, migraines and acne. My mother took me to her gynecologist and there I was prescribed the pill. I didn't ask many questions about it, because it was the only solution to my problems and secretly it made me feel like a real woman.

I was a late bloomer. But thanks to the pill, I got bigger breasts and my skin looked better. I gained more self-confidence. I didn't know any better then and didn't realize that hormonal contraception was going to have so many drawbacks for me. Over the years, I tried every form of hormonal contraception. The pill, the vaginal ring, a copper IUD, a hormonal IUD, you name it. Every time, I didn't feel a hundred percent comfortable with it. And yet there was no other direction for me, as I wasn't aware of any other options. If I had had the information then that I have now, my life would probably have been completely different. It was only in 2016, the year I got married, that I found out I had PCOS. Polycystic ovary syndrome (PCOS) is one of the most common hormonal disorders in girls and women. It would be tough to get pregnant, I was told, but the doctor would look at this the moment I decided to start trying to have children.

I'm not the only one who has PCOS, by the way. As many as 4 to 20 percent of menstruating women worldwide have this hormonal disorder. Some 25 percent of women have multiple cysts on their ovaries, but that does not necessarily mean you have PCOS. To get that diagnosis, you must meet at least two out of the three symptoms.

- Normally, each ovary has three to ten follicles. In PCOS, more than twelve follicles per ovary can be seen on an ultrasound.
- The hormonal balance in the ovaries is disrupted and you produce too many male hormones, which can cause acne and excessive hair growth.
- As a result, you may experience no or less frequent ovulation with an irregular cycle, or no menstruation at all.

And then suddenly, six months after my PCOS diagnosis, I turned out to be pregnant. How was that possible? The doctors had told me that it would be difficult to get pregnant ... And there I was, completely in shock. I am someone who likes to plan things. Just six months before, I was crying because I thought I was infertile and now I was crying because it turned out I had an unplanned pregnancy. In hindsight, I was very grateful because I realize that many women struggle to get pregnant, including women with PCOS.

Luckily, my pregnancy and delivery went very smoothly, and in February 2018 I gave birth to a healthy son, Richard. After my pregnancy, the doctor advised me to have a hormonal IUD inserted. 'That will be easiest for you, because you'll hardly have any bleeding and you are also protected against an unplanned pregnancy," the doctor said. 'Ok, let's go for it,' I thought. But after one and a half years, I was back at the gynecologist, once again with tears in my eyes, because my skin was so inflamed and covered in acne, making me feel like I was fifteen again.

The acne was the result of the hormonal spiral, I was told. It is apparently a common side effect; more than one in a hundred women experience it and I was one of them. The solution was to take the pill in combination with the IUD to make the acne disappear. What? I was so desperate that I gave it a chance, but after two months I noticed little to no improvement. Moreover, it went against everything I really wanted. I decided to have my hormonal IUD removed, stop taking the pill, and look for other solutions.

In that search, I discovered Sensiplan, a natural contraceptive method. You learn to track your cycle based on various body signals, such as your basal body temperature and uterine and cervical mucus.
It is a scientifically based way to determine your fertile days. A new world opened up for me. I also completed an additional course in Nutrition & Fertility at Monash University in Australia, because a healthy cycle also means a fertile cycle.

My first discovery was that a cycle consists of different phases and that your body has different needs during each phase. Various terms are used to describe these phases, but I prefer to compare them to the four seasons: autumn, winter, spring and summer. During each season, your body has different needs.

The clearest phases are autumn, the phase before your menstruation, and winter or your menstrual phase, the phase in which you bleed. Those are, as you may have already experienced yourself if you have a natural cycle, definitely not the periods in which you are bursting with energy. Quite the opposite. On those days, we prefer to get under a blanket with a box of chocolates, a warm cherry pit pillow, and a romantic movie. You may also have noticed that at other times of the month, after your period for example, you have much more energy. Then you're in spring and summer of your cycle.

The fluctuation in your emotions and energy that you may experience is due to the hormones that change throughout the month. These hormones, if you are not pregnant, eventually help your body expel the unfertilized egg every month. Every month, your body prepares for pregnancy, whether you want to have children or not. If your egg cell is fertilized, then you are pregnant. If it is not fertilized, it is expelled from your body through your uterine lining, or endometrium. Your hormones are in charge of this entire process of ovulation, from building up the endometrium to menstruation.

They not only regulate your menstrual cycle, but also have an impact on your overall physical and mental well-being. Your hormones affect, for example, your appetite, your ability to concentrate, and your energy level. They also ensure that physically at one moment you can do a lot, and the next you need more rest. It is normal for you to feel different throughout the month and maybe even experience a mood swing (or two or three). You can read more about how hormones work in this book, starting from page 51.

I first learned to recognize the phases of the cycle in myself about five years ago. During my autumn I felt lonely, my winter was a 'bloody hell', while in spring and summer I felt recharged and amazing. I also found out that I could better manage my menstrual aches and pains by, for example, taking more rest when I had a lot of symptoms. Thanks to small adjustments in my lifestyle combined with the right dietary supplements, I started noticing a positive difference in my cycle. That didn't happen overnight, but gradually I saw results. I felt better, more stable, and my acne disappeared.

I continued to deepen my knowledge of the subject over the years. My main sources of inspiration are Dr. Stacy Sims, PhD, an expert in female physiology, Dr. Jolene Brighten, an expert in female health and hormones, and Nicole

Jardim, certified Women's Health Coach and author of *Fix Your Period.* Stacy Sims shows that in sports, it is still often thought that women should train like men, with the same training schedules and principles. That is of course nonsense, since we have a very different hormonal cycle and other needs. Dr. Jolene Brighten focuses on quitting the pill with her bestseller *Beyond the Pill*, while Nicole Jardim has helped many women address hormonal issues with the right supportive nutrition and activities. These women are all experts who dare to view the cycle from a completely different, female perspective.

Their insights encouraged me to take my journey a step further. I also wanted to help other women with that knowledge. Because everyone has the right to have a healthy cycle, whether you have a desire to have children or not. And so Guud Woman was born, a company that my husband Jan and I started to help women feel good every day of the month. We do this by sharing our knowledge, offering chat support with experts, and developing our own line of natural dietary supplements.

In addition to a new 'professional' baby, I was also personally ready for a second baby, after living according to my cycle and using Sensiplan for four years. This time I wanted to take a more deliberate approach. I kept all my data in an app, *Natural Cycles*, which allowed me to accurately predict when to expect my ovulation. Because even though I am now an expert in the field of the menstrual cycle, my own cycle remains a challenge with a fluctuating duration of 35 to 55 days due to PCOS. A real challenge to get pregnant, indeed. And yet, it worked. In July 2022, when I was fully immersed in writing this book, I found out that I was pregnant with my second child. I was once again so grateful.

With *Decode Your Cycle*, I want to inspire you to live according to the four seasons of the menstrual cycle. Since I have discovered that a menstrual cycle is so much more than just having your period, a whole new world has opened up for me. I was able to recognize patterns, I discovered where those intense mood swings came from, and why my skin had more breakouts in certain weeks of the month. Or even how my self-confidence and libido varied throughout my cycle. I hope you and many other women will join me in learning to use the benefits of the cycle, because once you are aware of it, it's the best compass possible to navigate through your life.

> Life is not linear, it is cyclical. Break free from limiting beliefs and honor each phase of your menstrual cycle, whether healing, resting, growing or thriving.
>
> UNKNOWN

EXPERTS

Because there is still much to be done in the field of women's health and a lot of research is lacking, I find it important to surround myself with experts who also delve into this subject. In this book you will notice that I consulted with a number of progressive women, such as gynecologist Joke Bulthé, doctor Annaïk Van Branteghem, fysiologist Colette Peeters, midwife Rebecca Verhofstede, Sarah Ahannach (PhD), hormonal coach Bénédicte De Jaeger, Certified Women's Health coach Nicole Jardim, skin expert Marion Naudts, sexuality and relationship coach Leen Scholiers, nutrition expert Lily Joan Roberts, and hormone coach & personal trainer Axelle Wilssens.

I thank these women for shaping this book and sharing their knowledge and insights. I am very grateful that I have been able to surround myself with them in this phase of my life.

Rebecca Verhofstede
Rebecca graduated as a midwife in 2008 from Artevelde University of Applied Sciences in Ghent, Belgium. In 2010, she obtained a Master's degree in Health Education and Promotion from Ghent University. Triggered by her final project and motivated to do something new, she started a doctoral research in Social Health Sciences at the Free University of Brussels and Ghent University. She successfully defended her four-year research project in November 2015 and obtained her degree. Since the birth of her eldest daughter, she has started to delve into the subject of fertility, and helps women chart their cycles using the Sensiplan method. That way, she has already guided several women and couples in the natural and reliable avoidance of pregnancy or the fulfilment of their desire to have children.

Joke Bulthé

Dr. Dr. Joke Bulthé is a gynecologist and fertility expert in a multidisciplinary practice in Belgium and is affiliated with the University Hospital of Ghent. You can consult her for general gynecology and obstetrics, reproductive medicine, and functional-aesthetic gynecology.

She attaches great importance to individually mapping the menstrual cycle. Every woman learns to know her body better, feel how long each phase lasts and what effects the hormonal fluctuations have on the body. If you know which phase of your cycle you are in, you can take action to alleviate the symptoms and live accordingly.

Colette Peeters

Osteopath Colette Peeters (D.O., Msc.) runs a multidisciplinary group practice in Belgium, where she mainly focuses on patients with endometriosis, infertility, and gynecological and obstetric complaints. She has been conducting research for years on the effect of internal osteopathic techniques in sexually active endometriosis patients with chronic pain and dyspareunia (pain during penetration). Furthermore, she actively works on breaking the taboo surrounding this topic by giving interviews in various newspapers. Together with fertility doctor Wim Decleer, she made a podcast about endometriosis, which was set up by the Dutch broadcasters VPRO and NPO, and Belgian Radio 1. Colette Peeters has been an international teacher at the International Academy of Osteopathy for 22 years.

(For more information, visit: www.osteopaatcolette.be/en/)

Sarah Ahannach

Sarah Ahannach, PhD, obtained her master's degree in Forensic Biomedical Sciences at the University of Leuven and subsequently started as a doctoral researcher at the University of Antwerp, where she co-founded the *Isala citizen science* project. She is passionate about women's health and primarily conducts research on the female microbiome and is committed to science communication. Furthermore, she investigates the use of the microbial fingerprint in cases of sexual violence.

(For more information, visit: www.isala.be/en/)

Annaïk Van Branteghem
Dr. Annaïk Van Branteghem graduated as a primary care physician from the University of Ghent in 2017. In addition to her training as a primary care physician, she specialized in sports medicine and pursued additional training in non-surgical aesthetic medicine. To this day, she still pursues other courses in lifestyle medicine and preventive medicine. She has a passion for women's health and always pays attention to the complete picture with her patients.

Lily Joan Roberts
As a coach, Lily guides you on a healing path towards optimal health, energy, and mental clarity. Lily believes that health starts in our gut. When your gut is in balance, everything works better - including your menstrual cycle. Lily knows exactly how your gut influences your hormones, and she unravels how nutritious and delicious meals can add value to your health and well-being. Her background as a plant-based chef ensures that taste is central, her education as a herbalist represents her passion for the healing power of nature, her knowledge of Ayurveda nuances her emphasis on a holistic approach, while her title as a functional nutritionist sheds light on the impact of food on the body and mind.

Bénédicte De Jaeger
Bénédicte is a Hormone Health Coach and supports women who experience hormonal and premenstrual complaints, such as PCOS, thyroid disorders, irregular or absent menstrual cycle, migraines, bloating, acne, mood swings... and this based on lifestyle advice. You can also turn to her if you want to stop taking the pill or prepare your body for a healthy *pregnancy*.

Leen Scholiers
Leen is a sexuality and relationship coach. In addition, she is an internationally renowned hatha yoga teacher. In her coaching, she helps people connect with their bodies, experience more and better orgasms, and lead a life full of pleasure and happiness.

According to Leen, embracing sexuality not only brings more pleasure, but also general well-being and a sense of connection, and even meaning in life. This is because sexual energy is life energy that unleashes self-confidence and power, enabling people to fulfill their dreams.

As a relationship coach, Leen guides couples who are stuck (sexually) or even considering divorce, to rediscover each other as lovers and lifelong partners.

Marion Naudts
Marion has completed a training as a herbalist with a specialization in natural cosmetics. She continued taking courses and completed an additional two-year training as a herbalist at the European Academy for Natural Healthcare, a course in aromatherapy, and a training as an organic skincare formulator.

Since 2017, she has been the driving force behind *Marion maakt* and gives workshops on how to make natural cosmetics. In addition, she wrote two DIY books and launched her own line of natural cosmetics.

Axelle Wilssens
Axelle is a hormone coach, personal trainer and orthomolecular therapist. With a holistic approach and a focus on nutrition, lifestyle and supplementation advice, she guides women who struggle with hormonal complaints such as PCOS, PMS, irregular or absent menstruation, hormonal migraines and acne. You can also turn to her for intestinal problems, fatigue and food intolerances. In addition, she also guides women in achieving their fitness goals, such as fat loss, muscle building, gaining weight and getting stronger. This can be done separately or combined with addressing hormonal complaints.

Nicole Jardim
Nicole is a certified women's health coach, author, speaker, mentor, and founder of the Fix Your Period Collective. This unique membership program empowers women to reclaim their hormonal health through a science-based method that makes complex information accessible and engaging. Her work has positively impacted the lives of tens of thousands of people around the world.

CHAPTER 1

How to live according to your cycle

CHAPTER 1

How to live according to your cycle

Living in sync with your cycle may sound complicated, but it's not. I plan much of my life around my cycle. It may sound exaggerated, but I keep the phases of my cycle in mind in everything I do. In fact, now that I am pregnant while writing this book, I am a bit lost and missing the four seasons of my cycle to make better decisions. Believe me, it's worth a try. Your body and hormones will thank you.

What do you need to live according to your cycle?

- A natural cycle: this is what you have when you don't use artificial hormones like the pill, a vaginal ring or a hormonal IUD.
- A notebook or app to track symptoms such as mood, libido, sleep, cravings, cervical mucus...
- A thermometer to measure your basal body temperature.
- Patience and a little discipline for self-observation.
- Joy to embrace your body and cycle.

DISCOVERING YOUR OVULATION

The concept of living in harmony with your natural cycle, known as "The Cycle Syncing Method®" was introduced by hormone expert Alisa Vitti, author of WomanCode and In The Flo. These two books have completely changed my life. One of the lessons I learned from Alisa, and which was a real eye-opener, is how to live according to your cycle. It is a lifestyle where you fully connect with who you truly are. That may sound a bit woo-woo, but it's not. This way of life is based on your hormones, which control pretty much everything in your body, including your mind and energy.

By following the rhythm of your cycle, you become more aware of the unique needs of each phase and respond to them accordingly. Living in harmony with your cycle allows you to embrace your natural rhythm, helping to relieve symptoms like chronic stress, burnout, PMS, heavy periods, and mood swings.

How do you do that in practice, live according to your cycle? By tracking your cycle, and more specifically your ovulation. The peak of our menstrual cycle, which in fact is what everything revolves around, is ovulation, the moment when a mature egg is released from the ovary. The mature egg leaves the follicle and is taken up by the fallopian tube. An egg cell remains fertile for about 24 hours after ovulation. Fertilization occurs in the fallopian tube when a sperm cell has managed to get that far. If there is no sperm ready to fertilize the egg, the body rejects the unfertilized egg, along with the built-up endometrium. And so you get your period. Before that whole process, our body prepares itself every month. If you stop and think about it, you realize what an amazing machine the female body is, right? Read more about it as of page 42.

If you want to learn to live according to the seasons, I recommend to track your cycle so that you know when your ovulation takes place, because a healthy cycle is a fertile cycle. Hormonal contraceptives work by suppressing ovulation, with the pill being a prime example, as it completely prevents ovulation. The bleeding you experience during the pill-free week isn't a true menstrual period but rather a withdrawal bleed. As a result, you miss out on many phases of the natural menstrual cycle. By taking artificial hormones daily, you block your natural hormonal patterns and suppress your ovulation, so you won't get pregnant. Furthermore, artificial hormones can have side effects that we are often not aware of (see p. 148). Not that the pill only brings disadvantages with it. It remains a reliable contraceptive method that is still often prescribed by gynecologists. But it is also important to inform yourself well about which contraceptive method suits you as well as the advantages and disadvantages of each method. Do you take the pill because you have a difficult menstruation, an irregular cycle, severe cramps or acne? There are other options. The pill relieves your symptoms, but does not solve the underlying cause.

What happens now in concrete terms during such an ovulation? As a fetus of about five months, we as women have the largest number of potential eggs in our entire lives, around seven million. When we are born, there are 'only' two million and at the first menstruation in puberty, there are still 400,000 left. The egg cells are stored in follicles or vesicles and wait in the ovaries. During the first half of your cycle (the follicular phase), a number of follicles start to mature. The so-called follicle cohort emerges curious, as if to see if they are not going to miss the party. Only one of the follicles matures completely and embarks on the great adventure: ovulation. The ovary in which ovulation occurs can vary from cycle to cycle, as can the timing. Often it is thought that ovulation, and therefore the fertile period, occurs exactly in the middle of your cycle. In many biology books, the fourteenth day of the cycle is often referred to as the day of ovulation, but that usually deviates. With a short cycle, ovulation often occurs very early, sometimes as early as the eighth, ninth or tenth day. During long cycles, it can even take several weeks and occur at a time when you would actually expect your next period again. Eventually, the egg cell travels to one of the fallopian tubes and remains fertilizable for 24 hours for a potential encounter with a sperm cell. The remaining follicles shrink and disappear.

YOU HAVE MORE CONTROL OVER YOUR CYCLE THAN YOU THINK

Do you have control over how your cycle progresses? Actually yes, more than you think. Not only your age, but also your lifestyle has an impact on the quality of the egg cells. Some studies show that your eating habits can play a role in maintaining the quality of your egg cells.

The healthier your egg cell and follicle (egg sac), the better the hormones estrogen and progesterone can be produced. These are important for a healthy menstrual cycle. Midwife **Rebecca Verhofstede** says: 'Egg cells undergo various changes over a period of three months to prepare themselves for a possible ovulation. During this time, the genetic material is being copied and there must be absolutely no errors, as this determines the quality of the egg cell.

The hormones present in your body, your diet, the blood and oxygen supply, the amount of cellular energy produced, and stress all have an influence on the maturation of the egg cell and therefore on its further quality. The greatest effect of adjusting your diet, addressing stress, and taking supplements on egg cell quality is achieved when you have been working on it for at least three months.

You won't see immediate effects when you change your lifestyle, but after three months you should start seeing results and, for example, experience fewer complaints if you had any. Throughout the seasons, I will give you a guide on what foods are good for each phase. You can also read more about the impact of stress as of page 76.

If we were to depict the maturation of the egg cell and ovulation in a drawing, it would look like this:

FROM EGG MATURATION TO MENSTRUATION

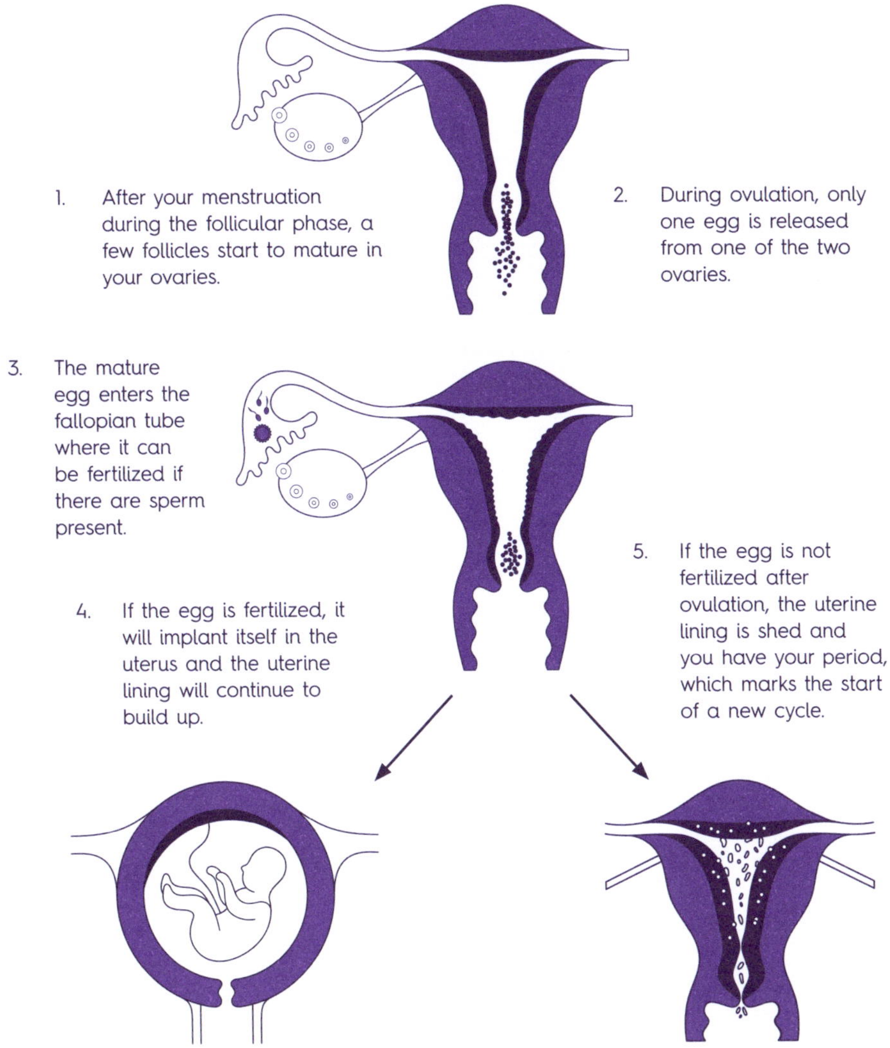

Tracking your ovulation or egg release lies at the heart of getting to know your body. It is useful because this way you can learn to live according to the four seasons of your cycle. First and foremost, you know what to expect, and when, from your body and mind. When we talk about the menstrual cycle, we often only think about the days when a woman is bleeding. They are usually experienced as dirty and miserable. When you ovulate, you usually have a lot of energy and you feel good. If you are aware of your body and your cycle, you can prepare and make the most of each phase.

You can also learn to interpret your body's signals **to avoid pregnancy** by tracking your basal temperature and monitoring changes in your cervical mucus. The consistency of your cervical mucus changes throughout your cycle, providing valuable insights into each phase (and indicating whether you're fertile or not). You might sometimes notice a wet spot in your underwear. Sometimes it is white, sometimes transparent, sometimes there is a lot of mucus and sometimes little. It is part of you and your amazing body. Whatever you call it, all of it is mucus that is produced by your cervix. It protects your uterus from intruders, but also tells you a lot about your cycle and your health.

Finally, tracking your ovulation is also helpful if you're **trying to conceive**. Ovulation is actually the ideal time to enjoy some intimacy.

What happens to your eggs when you take the pill?

Hormonal contraceptive methods such as the pill, the vaginal ring, or the hormonal IUD suppress your ovulation. That means that while eggs do mature in your ovaries, they do not reach their maximum growth and are not released from the ovary to be fertilized. The matured eggs do not survive. They die off and are then absorbed by the body. So you don't build up any extra stock of eggs when you take hormonal contraception.

HOW TO TRACK YOUR OVULATION

Figuring out your fertile days and ovulation isn't so hard, right? Ovulation always happens exactly in the middle of your cycle, doesn't it? Unfortunately, ovulation doesn't always occur halfway through your menstrual cycle. The moment of ovulation can vary from woman to woman and from cycle to cycle. The phase when your egg matures can last from the eighth day after the start of your cycle to when you are almost expecting your period. If you track only your menstruation, you can never be sure when you ovulate.

How do you know when you are ovulating? The best way to calculate this is to map out your cycle using the symptothermal method, such as Sensiplan. With this method, you learn to observe and map various body signals, so that you can determine your fertile and infertile days reliably using specific calculation rules. That helps you to identify your ovulation or egg release.

1. **Your basal body temperature is elevated.** If you measure your temperature daily at approximately the same time, in the morning before getting up, and have had enough sleep, your temperature can rise by 0.2 to 0.6 °C up to two days after ovulation. This is done by the hormone progesterone.
   The temperature remains high and drops just before or during the next menstruation back to the lowest temperature level. Please note that ovulation can sometimes occur without a rise in temperature. Therefore, it is recommended to analyze two or three cycles to accurately track your ovulation.

2. **The texture of your cervical mucus changes.** In the lead-up to your ovulation, your cervical mucus is stretchy and/or transparent. By checking the texture of your cervical mucus daily, you can predict an upcoming ovulation. Below we will tell you more about your cervical mucus.

3. **Your cervix changes.** The firmness, degree of opening, and position of your cervix change throughout your menstrual cycle. As your ovulation approaches, your cervix will open more, become softer, and rise higher.

As I mentioned above, your cervical mucus changes during your cycle. In the lead-up to your ovulation, the quality of your cervical mucus increases, allowing sperm to survive better and reach the egg more easily.

See the discharge on those days as a train on which the sperm cells can hitch a ride, all the way to the egg cell. But since you can't get pregnant for the entire month, this cervical mucus changes after your ovulation.

CERVICAL MUCUS

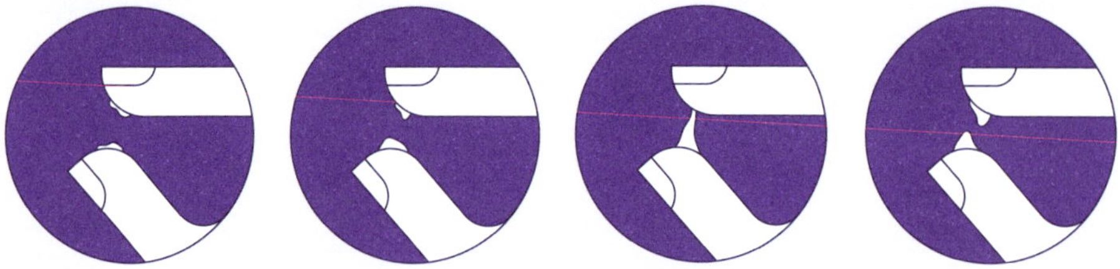

WINTER	SPRING	SUMMER	AUTUMN
Little or no discharge during menstruation	After your menstruation, when estrogen increases, your cervical mucus can be creamy, milky and sticky	During your ovulation, your cervical mucus is very stretchy and transparent	Before your period, your cervical mucus may be less, yellowish, granular and a bit thicker again

- **During your menstruation.**
  During your menstruation, you have less estrogen and progesterone. Less estrogen means less discharge. During this period, you have little or no discharge. If you already had discharge, you wouldn't be able to see it now because of the bleeding.

- **After your period.**
  Shortly after your period, you may observe little to no cervical mucus. Maybe your vulva also feels dry. As your estrogen increases, you will notice clearer cervical mucus: thick, sticky, milky, creamy or white. When it has dried, you will see a grainy layer in your underwear.

- **Around and during your ovulation.**
  You are about to ovulate and now see a clear difference in your discharge. Your vulva may feel wetter and you may notice stretchy and/or transparent cervical mucus on the toilet paper or in your underwear. It looks a bit like raw egg white. You also have a lot of discharge and it may even leak from your vagina.

- **Before your menstruation.**
  After your ovulation, estrogen will decrease again and progesterone will increase. This will result in a decrease in the quality and quantity of mucus. Your cervical mucus becomes thick, sticky, white, yellowish or grainy again, and can even be absent on some days.

What do you need to measure your ovulation?
Not much! First and foremost a **thermometer**, but one with two decimal places after the comma (so for example 37.52 °C). A regular thermometer is therefore not sufficient. And furthermore, **an app** as a tool to collect all the data (or you can write it down in a notebook, that's also possible). These are my favorite apps:

- **Natural Cycles.** This app is the only one officially approved by the American Food and Drug Administration (FDA) as a contraceptive app. Natural Cycles measures your fertility based on your basal body temperature. The app claims to be 99 percent reliable if you use it perfectly. It predicts your ovulation and menstruation. The data becomes more accurate as you add more information. The ovulation does not always occur in the middle of your cycle, which means you can still get pregnant at a time when you least expected it. The accuracy of the app increases as you record more cycles. You don't have the discipline to measure your temperature daily? Natural Cycles also has a partnership with Oura. A ring measures your temperature, keeps track of it, and sends it to the contraceptive app.

- **Flo.** This app predicts your ovulation and fertile days based on your cycle data. These are data that you enter yourself, such as the length of your past menstrual cycles and certain symptoms such as cramps or mood swings.

- **Clue.** Thanks to this app, you can learn a lot about your body. If you haven't paid attention during sex education classes, this is perfect for you. Clue provides you with both menstrual and PMS predictions based on the information you enter. All your data is neatly stored in a clear overview that helps you easily analyze and view trends. Just like Flo, the app provides an indication of your fertile days.

Attention! It is not recommended to use Flo and Clue as a reliable form of contraception. They remain apps that make *predictions* based on an algorithm of when you ovulate and therefore are fertile. They do not require you to monitor your basic body temperature, making them less reliable. They are useful for getting to know your cycle. They provide a clear overview of when your menstruation starts, how long it lasts, and even how heavy it is on different days, along with other symptoms.

Keep track of your temperature for at least one to three months. This way you can recognize patterns and better understand when your ovulation is approaching. **Check your uterine or cervical mucus daily** to know how it looks during each phase. Check for yourself every day whether there is mucus by your vaginal entrance, in your underwear or on your toilet paper.

CAN YOU MENSTRUATE WITHOUT OVULATING?

How can you know that you have had an ovulation? If a woman tracks her basal body temperature daily and there is no slight increase in her cycle, it may indicate that she has not ovulated. If there is no elastic cervical mucus, it can also indicate a lack of ovulation. When no egg is released from your ovary during your menstrual cycle, we refer to this as anovulation. However, you can have bleeding without a preceding ovulation. In this case, it is usually breakthrough bleeding.

Anovulation is common during certain stages of a woman's reproductive life, such as in girls who have just started menstruating. In the first year after the first menstruation, it is not uncommon for girls to have anovulatory cycles.

It also often occurs in women approaching menopause. Women between the ages of forty and fifty are more likely to experience a hormonal shift, which can lead to more frequent anovulation.

It is also possible to have anovulatory cycles while you are fertile, and there are many reasons for this. Below are some possible causes. If you are concerned about having anovulatory cycles, it is best to consult your doctor.

- Polycystic ovary syndrome (PCOS). This refers to a condition in which a hormonal imbalance causes small cysts or underdeveloped egg-shaped follicles in the ovaries. It can also cause irregular menstruation, excessive body hair, oily skin, weight gain, depression and infertility. Some women may have PCOS without experiencing these symptoms and may not know they have the condition until they try to get pregnant. If you have been diagnosed with PCOS, ovulation tests can give misleading results, because women with PCOS can have a high LH concentration throughout their entire cycle. Ovulation tests determine your fertile days by measuring the increase in LH in your urine. Therefore, I have never used it to confirm my ovulation.

- If you are underweight or overweight, this can have an impact on your menstrual cycle. You are more likely to have an irregular cycle or not have your period because ovulation has not occurred.

- Excessive physical activity over a longer period, such as long-distance running, can also cause ovulation to stop. By reducing the intensity and training volume, you can restore balance to your body.

- Stress and anxiety. It is advisable to consult your doctor if you think that your stress levels are preventing you from ovulating.

- Some medications can affect ovulation, including contraception. Always check the information leaflet of all the medications you use.

Are you completely new to tracking your cycle and want to know more about it? Then let yourself be guided by a Sensiplan coach. Sensiplan is a sympto-thermal method of family planning.
(*For more information, visit: www.sensiplan.be*)

Did you know

- During ovulation, your cervical mucus helps sperm survive in your vagina and allows them to pass through the cervix more easily?
- Your cervical mucus works as a natural lubricant? Sex is easier, you get wet faster.
- The more estrogen the follicles produce, the more the cervical mucus changes. It becomes more liquid and increases significantly in quantity.
- Your discharge during ovulation can be ten to twenty times more than normal!

YOUR CYCLE AS A GUIDE

I am a fan of living according to the rhythm of my menstrual cycle. I use my cycle as a compass that guides me on the right path. So I can lead a life that suits me and consciously choose for balance.

My first pregnancy was unplanned. Therefore, after giving birth, I got a hormonal IUD on the advice of my doctor. But after a year, as you could read in the introduction, I started experiencing acne and severe mood swings again. Both had a big impact on my self-confidence and quality of life. The acne turned out to be a side effect of the intrauterine device. As a solution, I had to take the contraceptive pill on top of my hormonal IUD. It didn't feel right, so I decided to have my hormonal IUD removed.

A woman is only fertile for a few days each month, so why should I take artificial hormones daily? Thanks to Sensiplan, I started to delve into my natural cycle. Just like with Nouchka (see p. 153), my body needed some time to regain balance. By living according to my natural cycle, I discovered that a different feeling is central in each phase of my cycle.

Does that mean I have to strictly follow the different phases of my cycle every week? Absolutely not, there are no strict rules. It's more a matter of using your cycle as a compass, which makes you more aware of which phase you are in and what your body and mind need at that moment. I can make better decisions regarding nutrition and exercise, as well as in the areas of work and social contacts.

This is how I try, if possible, to manage my energy and time. In my winter, I try to rest as much as possible and plan as much me-time as possible. In spring and summer, I plan as many social activities as possible again, because then I feel full of energy and good about myself. During autumn, I will ask for more help around the house or arrange for takeaway meals so I don't have to cook and clean up. I go to bed on time and plan a self-care moment, like a massage or a warm bath, or I guiltlessly watch a movie with a tub of ice cream. Furthermore, during the autumn phase, I try to write down my negative feelings such as frustration, anger or sadness in order to create more distance from them. If I don't take into account what my body needs in each phase of my cycle or if I live too hard, my symptoms during the next cycle can sometimes be more severe.

WE ARE SIMPLY NOT MEN

Cyclical living ensures that I live much more consciously and don't just unconsciously go along with the cycle of men. Because yes, men also have a cycle.

Men and women are equal, but not identical. The difference lies in the hormonal cycle.

The male cycle is controlled by the hormone testosterone, which peaks and declines according to a daily rhythm. The hormone level is therefore much more stable in men. At night, men produce testosterone. The testosterone level rises to a morning peak around 8 o'clock in the morning. From that moment on, testosterone levels start to decrease again. Between 7 and 9 o'clock in the evening, the testosterone level reaches its lowest point. This happens every 24 hours again.

In women, the hormones estrogen and progesterone are particularly active. Under the influence of these hormones, the woman's egg matures in about a month, which creates a monthly rhythm.

GRAPH OF TESTOSTERONE LEVELS IN MEN

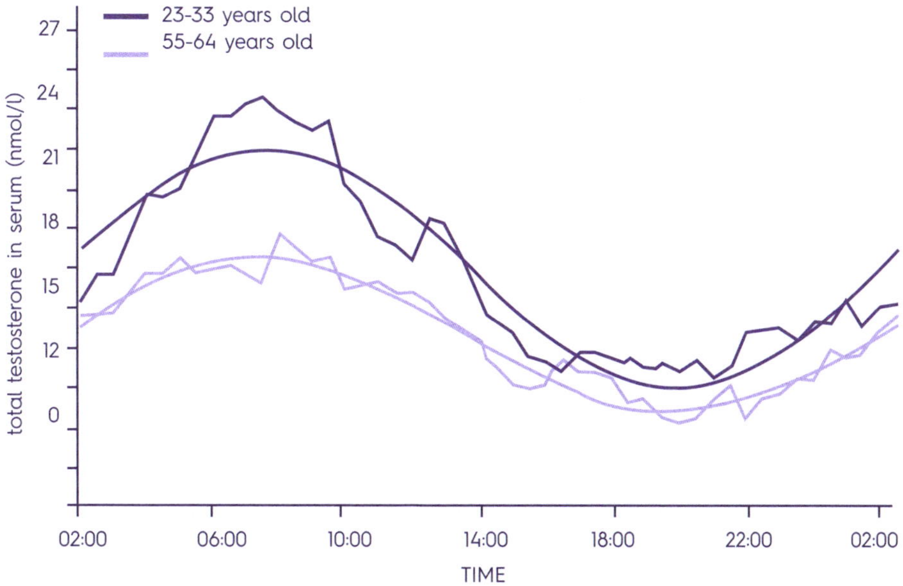

If we look at the rhythm of the male cycle, it is perfectly aligned with the daily work life and the day-night rhythm of the sun. The man is at his best during the day thanks to his cycle. Ideal for a standard nine-to-five workday. Especially in the morning, the testosterone peak provides energy, self-confidence, impulsiveness and temperament. For the rest of the day, there is enough testosterone left to stay cheerful and motivated. Afternoon is when the remaining amount of testosterone promotes productivity, focus and teamwork. And just when the testosterone level really drops and the man gets tired, the workday is over.

The woman's menstrual cycle lasts an average of 28 days, and you could say that we follow the rhythm of the moon, which makes us feel different every day. Some days we are full of energy, other days we want to take a step back. Women experience larger hormonal fluctuations. That affects how we feel and how we perform, but our society takes little account of that.

Men can also suffer from PMS

Everything goes well for men when they produce the right amount of testosterone every day, but if that doesn't happen, it can have many consequences. As men get older, testosterone production naturally decreases. Then a man enters the so-called andropause, the male version of menopause. The complaints associated with it occur much later in men than in women, around their seventies.

If a man temporarily produces less testosterone, it also has a name: Irritable Male Syndrome or IMS. There is little known about Irritable Male Syndrome (IMS) and only recently has this syndrome been studied. IMS can be caused by factors such as stress, poor nutrition, anxiety and depression. Sometimes it is also an empathetic response. If the partner's wife has, for example, PMS, then the man may also develop symptoms. He can be nervous and irritable, have a lower libido and a low sense of self-worth, be tired and struggle with concentration problems. IMS is more common than you think, so men should definitely not ignore such complaints.

YOUR CYCLE AND YOUR PRODUCTIVITY IN THE LABOR MARKET

Many women do not realize the extent to which their hormonal cycle can affect their energy levels and mood swings during the month. If we were to take the menstrual cycle into account more in the workplace, it would also provide added value to our productivity. Studies have shown that women experience a loss of work productivity due to their menstruation, averaging nearly nine days per year. Some 80 percent of women reported experiencing reduced work productivity due to their menstrual symptoms. I am shocked by such high figures. It is therefore high time to change this. By creating more awareness and sharing knowledge about the menstrual cycle, women can empower themselves in the workplace and beyond.

With this book, I want to inspire and teach women how to use their cycle to their advantage, and thus feel better and experience fewer symptoms. So women can be more empowered, and I am convinced that they will also radiate this to those around them and at work.

TESTIMONY

Natasha Casteleyn

(JEWELRY DESIGNER NIMZU)

In 2019, after intense years of carrying and giving birth to two children and starting my own business, my body called out that it was enough. I bled for months on end and the only 'solution' I got from the primary care physician and gynecologist was a prescription for the pill. I decided to take matters into my own hands and start tracking my cycle to investigate how it also affected my intense emotions. I began to recognize patterns that had been a blind spot both personally and professionally.

I am naturally very enthusiastic and a 'go-getter'. I would often come up with ideas for events or sales strategies, and in my impatience (hello, Aries) I would systematically plan their execution barely two weeks later. It started to become noticeable to me that at the moment of execution, my energy was extremely low and I actually wanted nothing more than to crawl under my duvet. Often this would lead to self-criticism and I would be disappointed in myself.
By tracking my cycle, I began to see that these phases coincided with my cycle and started taking them into account.

If I have all sorts of creative ideas now (often from day 4 to day 11), I plan their execution a month later to be at that same energy level. Often, I even let an extra cycle pass to see if the enthusiasm remains and to determine if it wasn't just a 'follicular inspiration' and perhaps not such a good business idea after all. That has made me much less reluctant to attend events or have contact moments with my clients.

Those observant among you will see that I am very active on Instagram (@ nimzu_) during the first ten days of my cycle. That's when I'm very good at clearly communicating my message. Two weeks later, I am much quieter and therefore you see me less often. In the past, I used to force myself to be visible online all the time, but because the energy wasn't right, it often didn't have the same effect. I am now letting go of that and focusing more on the work behind the scenes of my business during the last ten days of my cycle. Then I plan, for example, technical settings that can optimize sales. Or I work on administrative tasks that are often put aside during the follicular phase.

A recurring pattern that I have since identified is that towards the end of my cycle my critical voice emerges. 'What are you actually telling people online? Who cares about any of this? Is that relevant?' That doesn't always make it easy. Meanwhile, I allow that little voice, but don't give it too much attention. I know that I will be able to communicate confidently from my heart again a week later, regardless of how it is received by others.

In short, this is how I do it:

- WINTER: I try to incorporate enough moments of rest. If possible, I avoid appointments with clients, and make more time for swimming, going for a coffee, journaling and being alone.

- SPRING: I usually feel a vibrant energy. In spring, I have to restrain myself from being too loud and intense towards my team. I am full of energy and ideas. Often, I also want to change a pre-made schedule. Fortunately, I recognize that by now and I can openly discuss and put it into perspective with humor with my team.

- SUMMER: I am less focused on my business and feel that I want to connect more with my family. I want to go to the sauna, lie on the couch with the kids, romp and play together. My physical senses are sharper and the businesswoman is momentarily quieter.

- AUTUMN: the energy decreases, both mentally and physically. I turn inward a bit more. I reflect on the decisions and actions we took in the past weeks. I am more analytical. The critical voice gets louder. Just before I get my period, I often have a 'no bullshit day'. Certain things come to the surface that I have covered with the cloak of love during the previous phases. Those are the days when I express things that have been on my mind for a while: often less influenced by emotions, but more down-to-business and to-the-point.

The phrase that echoes throughout my entire cycle is: *'Don't let your summer woman be in charge of your agenda.'*

CHAPTER 2

How do we women function?

CHAPTER 2

How do we women function?

Before I take you through the four seasons of your cycle, I think it's useful to first touch on a few basics of the female body. Think of it as a brief recap if you remember your sex education or biology classes well, or a brief information session about your body if this is new to you. No worries, many women are not familiar with the correct terms when it comes to their own genitals, let alone where those parts are located. Unfortunately, it is typical for our society that we don't talk much about our bodies, especially not about our genitals, which is a big disadvantage when something is wrong. Do you always know exactly where you feel something then? The more knowledge you have about your body and yourself, the better you can explain to a doctor what feels normal to you and what does not. And the better you can make decisions that suit you. It is an opportunity to follow your gut feeling, which is sometimes necessary, as a doctor cannot feel what is going on in your place and can come up with an even better solution that truly suits you using your feedback. So, back to the basics, how does our body work again?

WELCOME TO WOMANHOOD
Can you name your female organs?

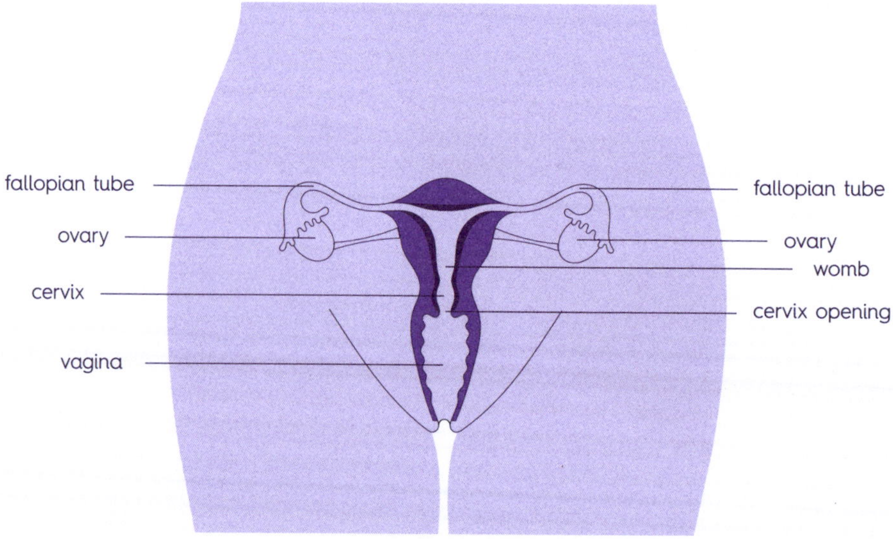

WOMANHOOD: A TIMELINE

FIRST MENSTRUATION	REPRODUCTIVE PHASE	PERIMENOPAUSE	MENOPAUSE
AGES 11-16	AGE 16-44	AGE 35-45	AGE 45-55
It usually starts with light bleeding. In the beginning, your menstruation can be irregular.	The most fertile phase in a woman's life is between the ages of 20 and 30.	This transitional phase causes changes in your menstrual cycle (shorter, longer, more irregular and/or heavier bleeding).	You are no longer fertile, your eggs are depleted, and you no longer menstruate.

THE WOMAN IN A TIMELINE

Life unfolds in stages. The reproductive phase of a woman starts from the first menstruation and ends with the last menstruation.

Your first period

In the two years before a teenage girl starts menstruating, a lot changes in her body. The hormones increase, her breasts grow and she gets pubic hair. The first menstruation (menarche) is one of the most important subsequent phases in puberty. The average age at which girls have their first menstruation is between 11 and 16 years old.

When girls first start menstruating, their cycle is different from when they are further along in their reproductive phase. Menstruation is not immediately regular after the first time. Sometimes a second menstruation can be delayed for a few months. During the first cycles, ovulation usually does not occur yet. Only from eighteen months after the first bleeding is there an ovulation. A menstrual cycle in teenage girls can sometimes last longer (on average 45 days) and can cause more blood loss or cramps. Only from their twenties onwards do most women have a regular menstrual cycle. From the moment a girl starts menstruating, her reproductive phase begins.

Did you know...

If you start menstruating for the first time at the age of twelve and enter menopause at the age of fifty, you will have menstruated for approximately five years of your life.

The reproductive phase

The reproductive phase is the phase in which we can reproduce (procreate). This is from the first menstruation until the last. This phase is also called the fertile age and lasts until about your forty-fourth year of life.

Between the ages of twenty and thirty, you are most fertile. The quantity and quality of your eggs decrease from the age of thirty. You are born with all the eggs you will ever have (one to two million immature eggs). From then on, a few eggs die every day.

During your reproductive years, about ten follicles grow each month per ovary. One egg matures completely. Only this egg will embark on the great adventure, namely ovulation. The other matured egg cells are expelled from the body through menstruation.

Your last fertile years: the perimenopause

During the last fertile years, a lot happens in your body. This phase leading up to menopause is called the perimenopause. Perimenopause literally means 'around menopause'. It is the phase in your life when your body starts preparing for menopause. It is sometimes also called the 'transition' and usually starts a few years before menopause actually begins. During perimenopause, your ovaries produce less estrogen and prepare to stop releasing eggs, but be aware that you can still get pregnant during this phase of your life. And this brings physical symptoms with it. For some women, it is also quite an emotional journey, as it signifies the end of their fertile years.

YOUR MENSTRUATION TELLS YOU ABOUT YOUR HEALTH

I thought in all those years before my PCOS diagnosis that it was normal for me to have so many symptoms. Pain and acne are just part of menstruation, right?

It may also seem like most women you know, including yourself, experience sensitive breasts, headaches, bloating, cramps, fatigue, acne and mood swings before their period, but this is not the norm. If you menstruate without PMS symptoms (see p. 93) that take over your daily life, it means that your hormones are 'happy'. You may experience certain complaints, but they should not disrupt your daily life. It is possible that you have a little less energy, experience mild cramps or notice a pimple every now and then, but if these complaints are painful and occur frequently, that is not how it should be. Of course, the pain threshold may vary from one person to another, and that is certainly a factor to take into account. But generally speaking, severe complaints are definitely not normal, also if they occur frequently. And so also not because we have had to hear for generations that they are just part of menstruation. They may indicate an imbalance in hormones, a hormonal disorder such as PCOS, endometriosis (see p. 174), adenomyosis, menorrhagia, pelvic inflammatory disease (PID), a uterine fibroid (fibroma), cyst on the ovary, or some other condition. If you feel that something is not normal, be sure to talk about it.

What is not normal?

- Adenomyosis or internal endometriosis (see p. 174) is a condition in which endometrial glands and stroma are found in the muscular layer of the uterus. This can lead to heavy menstruation, pain during intercourse, pelvic complaints, etc.
- Menorrhagia: heavy menstrual bleeding and is a medically recognized condition with physical consequences, such as fatigue, iron deficiency anemia and reduced immunity. This often indicates an underlying gynecological condition.
- PID: an inflammation of the pelvis is also called PID. This comes from the the English term pelvic inflammatory disease resulting from, for example, a sexually transmitted disease (STD) such as chlamydia or after an infection caused by a curettage/abortion

delivery. Abdominal pain is often the only symptom, but PID can also cause heavy menstruation and colored and odorous vaginal discharge.

- Fibroids, also known as myomas, are benign growths in or on the uterus. The exact cause of uterine fibroids is not precisely clear.
- A cyst on the ovary can be malignant or benign. A benign cyst can grow, but it does not spread. The cells from a malignant cyst can spread (cancer).

WHAT IS A 'NORMAL' CYCLE?

The frequency, length and intensity of your periods varies from person to person and from cycle to cycle. If your cycle doesn't sync up with that of your friend or sister, that's okay; as long as it fits your body. Did you know that it is actually a persistent myth that women's menstrual cycles synchronize? It was long believed that women who lived together always menstruated at the same time. That turns out to be absolutely incorrect. The famous study from 1971 that seemed to prove 'menstrual synchronization' has been debunked multiple times since then. Do yours and your friends' or sisters' happen at the same time? Then it's just a coincidence.

If you know what is normal and healthy for you, it becomes easier to notice when something is wrong. Over the years, I have discovered that many women do not know what a normal cycle is. But honestly? I didn't know it five years ago either. In school, we always learned that a cycle lasts 28 days and that you ovulate on day 14, halfway through your cycle. Nothing could be further from the truth. In reality, this only occurs in a minority of women. What is a normal cycle then?

1. **You have regular menstruation.**
   A normal cycle can vary between 22 and 40 days. This is a regular cycle. If you are above or below that, then you have an irregular cycle and it never hurts to contact your gynaecologist.

2. **Your menstrual blood is bright red.**
   Bright red menstrual blood without clots is what you want to have. This is what you get when there is sufficient blood flow in the uterus. Bright red blood looks the same as the blood that comes out of a wound.

The color of your blood does tell you, if you have a natural cycle at least and therefore do not use hormonal contraception, something about your menstrual health. The color and thickness of menstrual blood vary from person to person.

- Generally, it is **bright or slightly darker red**. At the beginning of your period, it is often thicker. Furthermore, an abnormal color says something about your menstrual health. The 'ideal' scenario is that your menstrual blood is clear to **dark red.**

- **Brown** menstrual blood can indicate old, oxidized blood that usually occurs at the beginning or end of your period. If you lose brown blood throughout your entire menstruation, there may be something else going on and it's best to discuss this with your doctor. Please note that women who are breastfeeding may also experience irregular brown bleeding.

- If your blood is **purple**, like frozen blueberries, that is a sign that you have too much estrogen. If your estrogen levels are much higher than your progesterone levels, this can also cause various menstrual problems, which you can read more about on page 48.

- A short menstruation with **light pink** loss can be a sign that your body produces little estrogen and therefore has difficulty ovulating. A low estrogen level can have various causes. It may be that you are not getting enough vitamins or nutrients because, for example, you are following a too strict diet or exercising too intensively. Another trigger is too much stress, so take good care of yourself and get enough rest! Discover more about how stress affects your cycle on page 76.

If you are concerned about the color or amount of your menstrual blood, it is wise to make an appointment with your primary care physician or gynecologist.

Six alarm signals in your cycle

1. **You bleed a lot or for a long time during your period.**
By bleeding a lot, I mean that you have to change your tampon, cup or pad every one or two hours, or that you menstruate for longer than a week. Normal blood loss is between 25 and 40 milliliters throughout the entire menstrual cycle, with a maximum of about 80 milliliters.

2. **Your blood loss (during a natural cycle) is not bright red.**
Dark, purple, gray or brown blood and the presence of clots can indicate poor circulation of the uterus. Blood stagnation in the uterus can cause pain. If you experience these symptoms, we recommend contacting a doctor.

3. **You are not getting your period at all.**
If you don't get your period (also known as amenorrhea), first rule out the possibility of being pregnant. Take a pregnancy test or get your blood tested. Aren't you pregnant? Then there is probably something else going on.

- Stress, being underweight or certain medications can cause you to stop menstruating.
- Breastfeeding can also cause you to have no or irregular menstruation. The hormone prolactin released during breastfeeding can cause you to have irregular or no periods. Your menstrual cycle will naturally return once you breastfeed less frequently or stop breastfeeding altogether.
- If you miss your period for several months in a row and also have other symptoms (such as acne, hair growth or hair loss, or if you gain or lose weight), chances are you have a hormonal disorder. To determine this, I recommend you visit your primary care physician or gynecologist.
- Women who stop using hormonal contraception sometimes have to wait months for their first period to return. Give your body time to restore balance. If your period still hasn't arrived after three to six months, it is advisable to make an appointment with your gynecologist as soon as possible.

4. **Your periods are irregular or occur frequently.**
   If your cycle lasts longer than forty days or if the length of your cycle varies more than seven to nine days per month, you may have an irregular menstruation. An irregular menstruation, or a long or short cycle, can have various causes, such as being overweight, weight loss, stress, hormonal imbalance, or a hormonal disorder like PCOS.

   If you are worried, it is wise to talk to your primary care physician or gynecologist. Note: breastfeeding can also cause irregular or absent menstruation, as your body produces different hormones that suppress ovulation. In that case, I wouldn't worry.

5. **You are experiencing breakthrough bleeding.**
   Breakthrough bleeding refers to spontaneous bleeding that occurs between two menstrual periods. This is also known as 'spotting'. There are many reasons why you may experience intermenstrual bleeding. It can be caused by hormonal imbalance or by the type of contraceptive you are using. It can also be an early sign of pregnancy. There are many possible reasons, from innocent or fun to a little scary (endometriosis, fibroids, polyps or even an STD). If you frequently experience bleeding between your periods, I recommend visiting your primary care physician or gynecologist.

   Some women also experience light bleeding around ovulation. An ovulation bleeding is usually short-lived and can be accompanied by pain. It can be the result of hormonal fluctuations around ovulation due to the sudden drop in estrogen levels.

- **You are experiencing painful cramps.**
  More than 60 percent of all women experience cramps. They occur because the uterine muscle contracts. It is not always possible to determine the specific cause. Often you get cramps because you have more of the hormone prostaglandin than normal. Prostaglandins are substances that are produced in the uterine lining and regulate many processes in the body, such as dilation and constriction of blood vessels, which prevents you from losing too much blood during your menstruation. They are

definitely useful, but having too much can make the cramps very painful. If you have so much pain that it affects your daily life, it is best to make an appointment with your primary care physician or gynecologist. Try to observe carefully if you have any other symptoms, as that can help determine the cause of your complaints.

If you experience a combination of the above symptoms, your hormones are screaming for attention and it's time to do something about it. If you have complaints, know that you can reduce your complaints with small adjustments to your lifestyle.

When do you visit a doctor?

- If you notice that your periods become heavier and/or more painful.
- If your menstruation lasts longer than seven days.
- If your menstrual symptoms are affecting your daily life.
- When you used to have a regular cycle in the past and it is now irregular.
- When you menstruate only once every three months or less frequently.

'SHE'S HAVING HORMONAL ISSUES AGAIN, RIGHT?'

Time for a short quiz! How well do you know your hormones and your body?

1. HOW DO HORMONES END UP IN YOUR BODY?

a. Through your food.
b. Your body produces them itself.
c. Through sunlight.

(b. Your body produces them itself.)

2. THE CYCLE BEGINS...

a. after the bleeding stops.
b. on the first day of bleeding.
c. on the day before the bleeding.

(b. On the first day of the bleeding.)

3. DO WOMEN HAVE DIFFERENT HORMONES THAN MEN?

a. Yes.
b. No.

(b. No)

4. FERTILIZATION OF AN EGG TAKES PLACE IN...

a. the ovaries.
b. the fallopian tubes.
c. the uterus.

(b. In the fallopian tubes)

How many did you get right? It was only when I started having 'problems' with my hormones that I began looking into it further. But actually it's quite strange that we know so little about it, don't you think? Hormones are actually the main actors in our body. They are like messenger substances that are produced in various glands of your body, for example in the head (in the hypothalamus and pituitary gland), the neck (in the thyroid and parathyroid glands), the abdomen (in the adrenal glands and in the pancreas), in the reproductive organs (in the ovaries and testicles) and in peripheral tissue such as breast tissue, fat cells, bones, skin and blood vessels. Your hormones and the organs that produce them are collectively called the endocrine system.

That has an impact on the functioning of our body. The hormones reach your organs and tissues through the bloodstream, where they then take control. An example: insulin regulates blood sugar levels, leptin regulates satiety, and cortisol ensures that we respond in stressful situations. Hormones are therefore the drivers of your body and regulate your menstrual cycle, your behavior and emotions, but also your growth and development.

The human body has about 100 hormones, and new ones are still being discovered. Everyone, both men and women, have the same hormones. Men also have female hormones (estrogens) and women have male hormones (testosterone). The quantities do differ. Depending on the hormone, you can measure the values through your blood, urine or saliva. A pregnancy test, for example, measures the presence of the HCG hormone in your urine.

Your female hormones and your emotions
Do you feel the same every day? I don't and you probably don't either. The different phases or seasons of your cycle are also controlled by your hormones. Because they fluctuate constantly and have such an immense impact, you can therefore feel different each time. If you are aware of this and take it into account in your daily life, you will feel more confident. You are prepared to make the right choices for yourself and your body. In this way, you live according to your cycle. That is a great opportunity to get closer to yourself. You bring out the best of your body and your life, every day.

Listening to your body is truly a challenge in our society. You have those days when you feel like you can conquer the whole world. Other days are tough, and early in the morning you already wonder how on earth you are going to get through the day. But in our society there is actually no room for an off day. If you don't feel well, you better get over it quickly, or have an extra coffee or a painkiller. Many women become overworked or feel stressed as a result. The typical 9 to 5 workday ignores our natural, female rhythm and is based on the daily cycle of men (see p. 35). Before starting my own company Guud Woman, I worked for a corporate company for seven years. It was a very masculine environment with fixed working hours from 8 am to 5 pm and a fixed lunch break. I was then still not living according to my cycle, but now that I think back, this rhythm didn't feel right for me. I experienced a lot of fatigue, cravings and headaches during that time. It was a period in which I drank a lot of coffee and survived on painkillers just to be able to perform well at work. Now that I work for myself (I understand that this may not apply to everyone), I can better set my boundaries. Mind you, in my case working for myself does not mean working less, but I can certainly work differently this way and I really like that!

There is no longer time in our society for days of rest and reflection. Because it will still take a while before we have changed the world, we might as well make ourselves as comfortable as possible in the meantime.

I have personally suffered from severe mood swings for years. Only when I started mapping out my cycle did I realize that my hormones played an important role in this. I don't want to blame them, but for years I thought there was something wrong with me. For most of my youth, I doubted my mental health. This also caused me to lose my confidence, relationships, opportunities and sometimes my faith in life, all because I didn't know what hormones are capable of.

That negative voice had such a big impact on my daily functioning that I didn't know what to do with myself until I started recognizing patterns by keeping track of my emotions and feelings in a mood tracker (like the Moody Month app). That way, I was able to discuss all sorts of things with the people around me. It also helped to write down my feelings and talk about them with my loved ones. By mapping my cycle and adjusting my lifestyle, my symptoms are no longer as severe. If all of this is very recognizable to you, then definitely seek help. Talk about it with friends and keep track of how you feel. Here is an example of how you can keep an emotion diary.

With this emotion diary, you can map out how you feel during certain moments in your cycle. It will help you to take a moment to reflect on your emotions and figure out if there is a pattern in your feelings.

EMOTIONAL DIARY

In the days before my period, I feel:

My energy level is:

At work, I feel:

On the love front, I feel:

On a social level, I feel:

On a mental level, I feel:

During my menstruation, I feel:

My energy level is:

At work, I feel:

On the love front, I feel:

On a social level, I feel:

On a mental level, I feel:

In the days after my menstruation, I feel:

My energy level is:

At work, I feel:

On the love front, I feel:

On a social level, I feel:

On a mental level, I feel:

What are the main female hormones?
Maybe you have already heard of the two most important hormones of your cycle: estrogen and progesterone. But there are more hormones that play an important role in your body and life; for example follicle-stimulating hormone, luteinizing hormone, testosterone, cortisol, insulin, prolactin ... All these hormones are produced in specific glands and tissues in your body, and each plays a part in your menstrual health and determines how you feel or perform. In this drawing, you can see how your hormones fluctuate according to the seasons of your cycle. For each season, you can read in detail which hormones have an impact. In the following, I will tell you more about the different hormones and their properties.

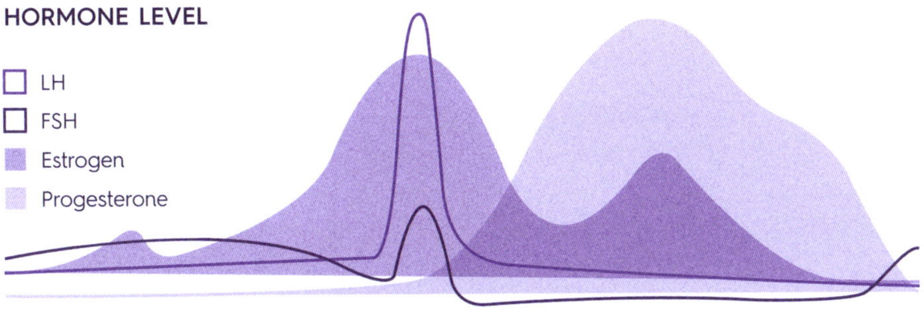

The four hormonal main characters of your cycle
There are four hormones that play the main role in the movie 'Your Cycle': estrogen, progesterone, FSH and LH.

1. **Estrogen**
   Estrogen is mainly produced in your ovaries in the maturing egg cells (follicles) under the influence of LH and FSH, but also in your adrenal glands and fat cells. The production only starts to pick up during puberty and it causes your breasts to grow, your uterus to develop, and your eggs to mature. Estrogen becomes the main player in regulating your menstrual cycle from that moment on and plays an important role in pregnancy. Estrogen is also responsible for strong bones, radiant and healthy skin, emotional stability, and good brain function. Estrogen plays a role in the production of serotonin and endorphins. Serotonin affects your mood, sleep, libido and eating behavior. Endorphins suppress pain and create a feeling of happiness. The correct balance of estrogen ensures that all your bodily processes run smoothly and that

you feel good in your own skin. The first few days after your menstruation, the estrogen level is still low. During the follicular phase (the week after your menstruation), estrogen levels rise again and reach their peak just before ovulation. This works as a trigger for the follicle-stimulating hormone. There are four types of estrogen.

When we talk about estrogen, we are mainly referring to estradiol, a form of estrogen that is most commonly found in women during their reproductive years. The other three forms are estrone, estriol and estetrol. Estrone is the main form of estrogen present in the body after the menopause. Estriol is an estrogen that increases during pregnancy. It makes the uterus grow and prepares the body for childbirth. Estetrol only occurs in pregnant women and is produced by the fetus's liver.

2. **Progesterone: helps your body prepare for fertilization**
   Progesterone is produced by the corpus luteum (yellow hormone-secreting body) and increases after ovulation. This hormone ensures that your body can prepare for fertilization by maintaining the uterine lining. It prepares your body for pregnancy and ensures a good blood flow to the uterus so that an egg can implant. During pregnancy (until about the 12th week), it ensures that your baby can grow well. When fertilization does not occur, the corpus luteum dies and the production of progesterone and estrogen decreases. This results in the shedding of the built-up uterine lining during menstruation and the start of a new cycle. A good progesterone balance helps maintain a stable blood sugar level and has a calming and stabilizing effect on your brain.

3. **Follicle-stimulating hormone**
   Follicle-stimulating hormone (FSH) stimulates the follicles. Those are the pouches in which the immature egg develops. That means that FSH helps your ovaries prepare your eggs. A number of follicles continue to develop, and after a while one follicle becomes 'dominant'. That grows into an egg and travels to the uterus. After FSH has done its job, the baton is passed on to the next hormone: luteinizing hormone (LH).

4. **Luteinizing hormone**
   The increase of luteinizing hormone causes the follicle to rupture and release the mature egg. From the ovary, the egg descends into the fallopian tube. This is what is referred to as ovulation. Your most fertile days coincide with this LH peak. The peak only lasts one or two days. Too bad, because the days around my ovulation I usually feel at my best. A deficiency of LH and FSH causes irregular menstruation in women, and sometimes the menstruation stays away completely.

   This can cause fertility problems. If you produce too little FSH, it will be more difficult to achieve ovulation. Insufficient LH is the cause of difficulty in maintaining your corpus luteum, which plays an important role in the production of progesterone.

The (essential!) supporting roles

- **Testosterone**
  This male hormone affects your libido. Women also produce this hormone (in the adrenal glands and ovaries), but in smaller quantities than men. Testosterone not only determines whether you have a sex drive, but it also stimulates body hair growth, muscle growth and sebum production. Greasy skin, acne, an increased libido, high blood pressure, interrupted sleep and insulin resistance can be caused by a high testosterone level. This is common in women with PCOS. Your testosterone levels decrease during prolonged stress. If you have a lot of stress, you usually don't have an excess of testosterone. However, you also don't want to have low testosterone levels either. A deficiency can lead to symptoms such as decreased libido, infertility, reduced muscle mass, hair loss, depression and energy dips. An important hormone to keep an eye on!

- **Cortisol**
  Cortisol is your main stress hormone. When you have a lot of stress, you make more cortisol. Your body then 'steals' progesterone, causing progesterone levels to drop. When that happens, it can mess up your hormones. It can lead to changes in the frequency and duration of your menstruation and make your menstrual symptoms worse every month.

- **Insulin**
  Insulin is produced in your pancreas and helps stabilize your blood sugar level. An unstable blood sugar level is an underlying cause of many hormonal problems and can have consequences for your menstrual health. It is important to keep your blood sugar level constant and avoid spikes. Your blood sugar level rises when you eat sugars.

  Sugars are converted into glucose. Insulin is then produced, because that hormone ensures that the glucose can be absorbed into your cells and does not remain in your blood. The more insulin you produce every day, the less sensitive the cells become to it. This is also called insulin resistance. Some of the glucose ends up in your liver, which converts it into glycogen.

  This is later converted back into glucose if your blood sugar level is too low. Think of it as a kind of backup. But if you eat too much sugar, you will overload your liver. And that is not ideal when your liver needs to break down estrogen after your ovulation phase. Discover on page 98 how you can support your blood sugar level and avoid energy dips during autumn.

- **Dehydroepiandrosterone (DHEA)**
  This hormone is formed from cholesterol and is produced in our adrenal glands, reproductive organs and brain. From DHEA, other hormones such as estrogen and testosterone are produced, which we need to allow our body to function properly. DHEA provides protection when your body experiences too much stress. When you're stressed, you produce cortisol. At the same time, DHEA is also produced, which controls the amount of cortisol. Once the production of cortisol becomes too high, DHEA can block this process. In this way, the negative effects of cortisol can be compensated for. Only with chronic stress can DHEA not function properly, and then less DHEA is produced.

- **Prolactin**
  Prolactin is a hormone that plays an important role during and after your pregnancy. It is produced by the pituitary gland, the small gland in your brain. Prolactin, together with oxytocin, promotes nurturing behavior, relaxation, deep sleep and stress reduction. The hormone

is mainly produced during the breastfeeding period. Prolactin is produced also outside of pregnancy and breastfeeding, but in much smaller amounts. Men produce a small amount of prolactin as well. The hormone suppresses ovulation, which often prevents menstruation in breastfeeding women. It's a clever trick of Mother Nature: as long as you're breastfeeding a baby, your body and mind are probably not quite ready for a new pregnancy.

But be careful: even though you may sometimes not have a period, it doesn't mean you can't get pregnant while breastfeeding.

HORMONE GLANDS

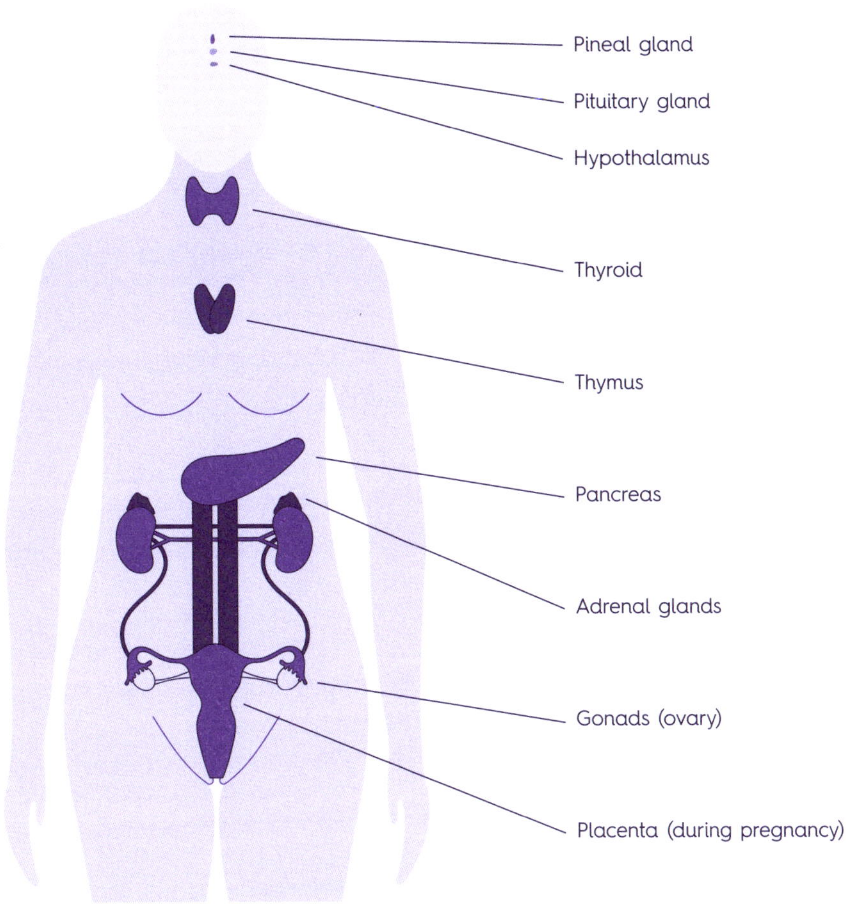

YOUR GUT AND YOUR CYCLE

Your gut health is responsible for your digestion, regulates metabolism, supports the immune system and provides protection against infections. In addition, it plays an important role for your hormones, which in turn are the main characters of the best movie ever: a healthy and fertile cycle.

Have you ever heard of your microbiome? Those are all the trillions of bacteria, yeasts, viruses and other single-celled organisms in your gut. It may sound a bit scary, but believe me, you need them. There are specific bacteria in the gut that are responsible for converting and eliminating estrogen from your body. If these bacteria cannot do their job, estrogen is reabsorbed into the body. When estrogen reaches its peak around ovulation, the excess is first broken down in the liver. The excess estrogen then leaves your body through your intestines and ultimately your stool. If you consume a lot of toxic substances such as alcohol, refined sugars and caffeine during that time of your cycle, your liver will prioritize them and estrogen will be put on the waiting list, so to speak. The hormone then enters the bloodstream and can cause estrogen dominance, resulting in various symptoms such as heavy menstruation, painful cramps, bloating, mood swings, acne and sensitive breasts.

Whether you eat meat or follow a vegetarian or vegan diet, there are a few tips that nutrition expert Lily Joan Roberts likes to share to keep your gut healthy.

1. **Drink enough water.**
   The ideal amount varies for each body, but approximately 1.5 liters is a nice average goal. Make it fun by alternating water with herbal tea or flavored water (add fresh lemon, mint leaves or cucumber).

2. **Eat all the colors of the rainbow.**
   Above all, enjoy the colors dancing on your plate! The more different colors, the better. They reflect the different types of vitamins and antioxidants that the food contains. This variety gives your body the diversity of the nutrients it needs. And the more natural sources of color and textures, the more fibers you consume. Fiber is important for smooth bowel movements.

Fibers are present in all plants, but can be found in large quantities in green leafy vegetables, nuts and seeds, whole grain products, and legumes such as beans, lentils and chickpeas.

3. **Reduce take-out meals.**
Most processed foods, ready meals and takeaways contain little fiber, are usually nutritionally unbalanced, often packed with preservatives and high in sugars. No time? Try cooking in advance and freeze meals. Preparing your own meals also gives your body more time to register what food is coming in, allowing it to trigger the right digestive juices. This allows you to digest more easily and absorb more nutrients.

4. **Chew well.**
This way, your body can absorb the food more easily and prepare your digestive system for processing the food. The more work is done in the mouth, the less work your stomach and intestines have to do. If you take your time to chew, your nervous system will also settle down.

5. **Fermented food.**
One of the simplest ways to keep your microbiome multicultural is by eating fermented food. That sounds exotic, but you probably already eat fermented food without realizing it. Some examples are chocolate, cheese, yogurt and wine, all the result of fermentation! But the real fermented stars are sauerkraut, miso, kimchi, kombucha and kefir. Fermented food helps the good bacteria in your gut and often contains natural probiotics. It has already been partially broken down by bacterial activity, making it easier to digest. It also contains a lot of extra vitamins, because sugar is converted into alcohol, acids and gases during fermentation. This provides a boost of vitamins B, C and K, antioxidants, useful enzymes and omega-3 fatty acids.

6. **Use as many herbs as possible.**
There is a complete first aid kit hidden in our kitchen! Herbs and seasonings such as onions, leeks, garlic, ginger and turmeric have anti-inflammatory properties and give your immune system a boost. They also contain a lot of vitamins. So do not underestimate what herbs and spices can do for your body. I really do recommend using them in large quan-

tities in your dishes for more flavor and health benefits! And you can also drink them: fresh thyme, cinnamon, fennel and mint provide perfect support for your digestion, gut and stomach.

7. **Avoid coffee and alcohol.**
   I know, this is really not what you want to hear. But coffee and alcohol often cause a drama in your gut, and therefore in your hormones. Coffee is likely part of your morning routine, but its high acidity can cause problems in your gut, lead to dehydration and put stress on your liver. Alcohol also keeps your liver too busy, so it doesn't have time to get rid of the excess estrogen, and this can cause a whole range of symptoms that you definitely don't want to deal with. You can alleviate menopause by following the rule:

   'Not at home, but only in a coffee bar if it is a really good cup of coffee.' So a coffee becomes a special treat instead of a habit. If you still drink that cup of coffee, always have a large glass (warm) water with it to compensate for dehydration. You can replace your coffee ritual with mindfully preparing matcha, or brew a chicory coffee. Enjoy a cocoa drink or make a chai latte.

8. **Be careful with stress.**
   It's easier said than done, but did you know that stress also affects your gut? It is not always avoidable, but if you feel stressed for weeks or months on end, it is time to do something about it. Unravel step by step what causes your stress and what you can change. Gradually integrate new rituals that bring you joy. Don't turn your life upside down in one go, because too much change at once can also cause stress! Read more about it on page 76.

9. **Mindful eating.**
   One of my great passions is becoming aware of how we eat, regardless of what we eat. Become aware of your habits and energy around meals and eating. One of the easiest ways to get your digestion back on track is by slowing down and relaxing more while you eat. Take your time and be grateful for the food on your plate. Focus on what you can add instead of what you are not allowed to do. The rest will follow naturally!

Your bowel movements and your menstrual cycle.

Maybe you have noticed it before. Just before or during your period, your bowel movements change. Some women experience constipation. Others, on the other hand, may have diarrhea. Whereas others don't have any problems at all. Whatever happens with your bowel movements, the changes often occur due to hormonal fluctuations.

After ovulation, just before your period, your progesterone level rises. This can cause food to move more slowly through your intestines, which can lead to constipation. If you suffer from constipation, then you know that it could be the cause.

As soon as your menstruation starts, the progesterone level decreases again. At the same time, the amount of prostaglandins increases. These are hormone-like compounds that regulate various things: they ensure that your uterus contracts (yes, cramps).

But they don't just stay in your uterus and can also end up in your intestines. This can cause diarrhea or make you have to go to the bathroom more often to empty your bowels.

How severe it is varies from woman to woman. Some may never experience a different bowel movement during their menstruation, or perhaps they are just never aware that their bowel movement is different during the various phases of their cycle. So besides tracking your mood, temperature and cervical mucus, you can now also monitor your bowel movements.

CHAPTER 3

Optimizing your cycle

CHAPTER 3

Optimizing your cycle

By learning about your cycle, you gain insight into how your hormones work. Cyclical living is therefore about listening to your body. Then you adjust your schedule accordingly. You can apply this in all aspects of your life, both at work and in your personal life. By adjusting your diet, exercise, stress regulation and sleep accordingly, you gain a lot of control.

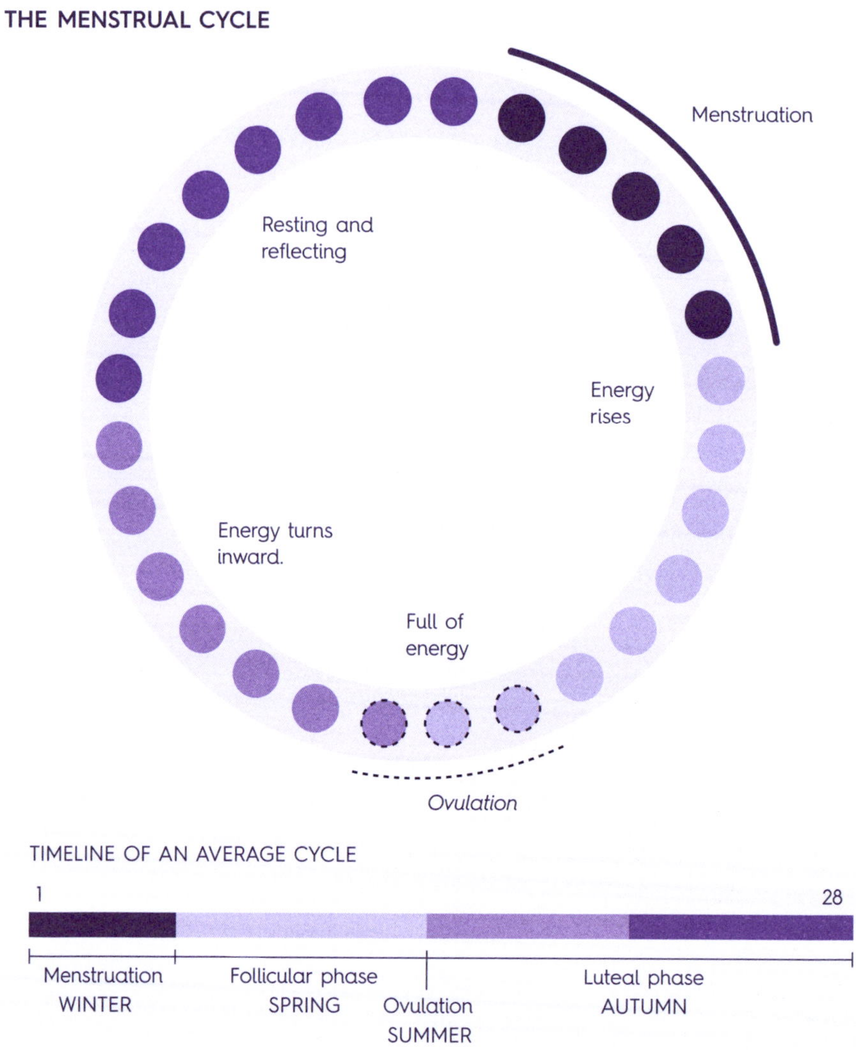

Your cycle consists of four phases. You can compare them to the four seasons. Every season has its ups and downs. You would think that autumn and winter are not fun, but the better you take care of your body in each phase, the easier it is for your body during autumn and winter. Get to know your cycle and use that knowledge to your advantage to feel good every day of the month.

The 4 seasons of your cycle

Winter.
The menstrual phase, the phase in which you lose blood. Winter begins on the first day of your cycle, which is also the first day of your menstruation. Your estrogen and progesterone levels are at their lowest. If you experience menstrual pain, be kind to yourself and take it easy. *Duration: 3 to 7 days.*

Spring.
After winter, you enter the follicular phase. The amount of estrogen starts to increase and the follicle-stimulating hormone (FSH) signals the start of your eggs developing. *Duration: 7 to 10 days.*

Summer.
The ovulation phase. The amount of FSH in your body increases even further, causing your ovaries to release an egg for the big adventure, also known as ovulation. Estrogen reaches its peak and helps thicken the uterine lining, so that a fertilized egg can implant later on. During this phase, you are most fertile. *Duration: 3 to 4 days.*

Autumn.
During the luteal (premenstrual) phase, progesterone plays an active role. If your body receives the signal that no egg has been fertilized, progesterone decreases and the built-up uterine lining is shed, about 12 to 16 days after ovulation. This is the beginning of your winter and the start of a new cycle. Your emotions are difficult to predict and you may experience negative thoughts during this phase. These common PMS symptoms are a result of strong hormonal fluctuations the days before your period. *Duration: 10 to 14 days.*

YOUR DIET AND YOUR CYCLE

We often tend to make the same dishes and buy the same products. I also catch myself doing this when I go grocery shopping and prepare food. Easy, right? But since I discovered that my cycle consists of four phases and that estrogen, progesterone and testosterone fluctuate during the month, I feel that my body needs different nutrients in each phase. Since I started adding specific vegetables, fruits, nuts and seeds depending on the phase I'm in, I feel that my body can support me better. Moreover, you create greater variety by eating differently every week. I also use my cycle to make better and more varied decisions in the supermarket.

The link between our gut and our hormones

According to nutrition expert Lily Joan Roberts, nutrition can have a big impact on your hormonal balance and how you feel. Did you know that your brain connects and communicates with your gut? This is called the brain-gut axis. It is crucial to your well-being and affects your productivity, mood, sleep, concentration and mental clarity.

A little fun fact: Some 95 percent of the feel-good neurotransmitter serotonin is produced in your gut, not in your brain!

Our hormones are influenced by the health of our gut and the microbiome. And if there is just one tool to get it healthy, it is your diet. Enough exercise, good sleep and sufficient relaxation all contribute to a healthy microbiome. But fresh and varied nutrition is the most important factor. Every day we enjoy different meals, and every particle of every ingredient that enters our bodies is processed and absorbed. The bacteria in the gut play an important role in digestion. They break down nutrients that the body itself cannot break down (see p. 60).

Sometimes we are not aware that some nutrients do more harm than good, such as antibiotics, alcohol, drugs, processed grains, trans fats, refined sugars, artificial sweeteners and colorings. Or we ignore intolerances, allergies or food sensitivities that can cause us to develop intestinal inflammation. Those inflammations can cause physical symptoms such as bloating, constipation, diarrhea, headache, muscle and joint pain, acne, but also mental problems, including depression, anxiety, concentration disorders and brain fog. They also disrupt your hormone balance, causing your sex, sleep, and mood hormones to become imbalanced.

It is clear that nutrition has a lot of impact on how we feel, and many studies are doing more research on this. By gradually adjusting your diet, you can already notice a big difference in your mood, focus and productivity.

Healthy eating can also be delicious: what is good for your body can also taste damn good! Once you start experimenting with herbs and different flavors, you will notice how much more interesting your meals become. Health and pleasure are a match made in heaven!

What we can consider as 'healthy food' is not a one-size-fits-all matter. The ingredients that work best for you depend on your personal microbiome composition, genetics and lifestyle. So: a diet that feels blissful for one person does not automatically work the same way for another.

Don't let this discourage you! Approach getting to know your body with a sense of curiosity. That also applies in the kitchen: experiment and try out different ingredients, flavors and dishes.

Doing things 'properly' doesn't mean you're going to restrict yourself with rules. Just enjoy the flavorful discovery process and keep in mind that nourishing yourself is a form of self-love. Listen to your hunger and satiety cues and remember the following: don't just fill up, but truly nourish yourself.

Don't be too hard on yourself and occasionally enjoy something that may not be so healthy. I think we all know that alcohol, caffeine, refined sugars and processed food are not ideal, especially not for your gut and hormonal balance. These ingredients can also cause more inflammation, which is best to avoid, especially the week before your period, as they will only worsen your symptoms. Also keep in mind that there is a sudden drop in estrogen and progesterone just before your menstruation. This hormonal change also causes more inflammation in your body, and combined with alcohol, caffeine, sugars and processed food you will then feel less well.

EATING ACCORDING TO YOUR CYCLE		MENSTRUAL PHASE (WINTER)
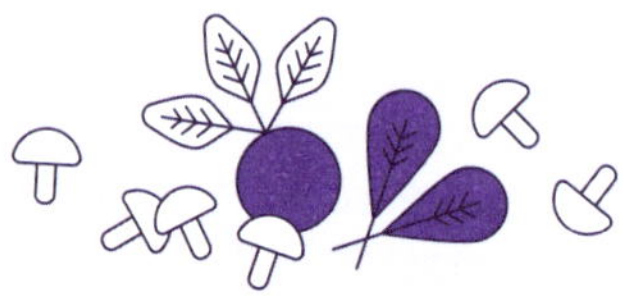	**VEGETABLES**	Kale Red beetroot Mushrooms Watercress Sweet potato Seaweed (kelp or wakame) Leafy greens
	**GRAINS**	Wild rice Brown rice Buckwheat
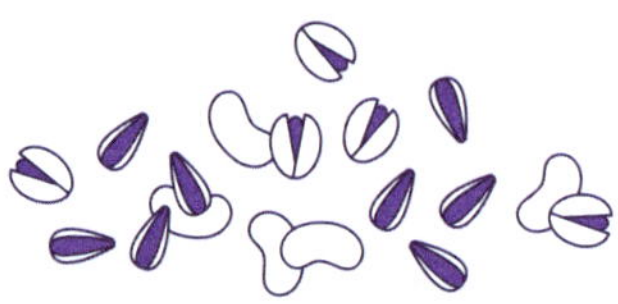	**NUTS & SEEDS**	Chestnuts Flax seed Hazelnuts Pumpkin seeds
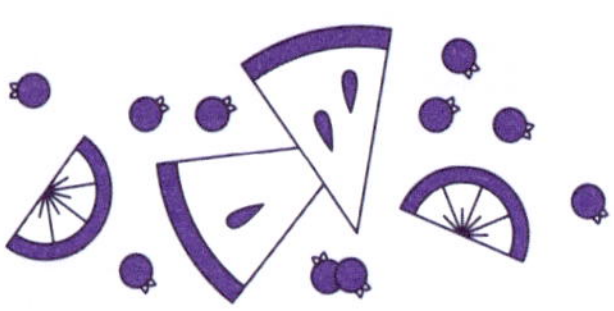	**FRUIT**	Blueberries Blackberries Watermelon Grapes Cranberries
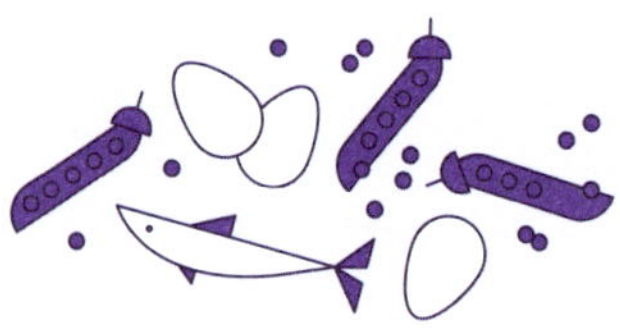	**PROTEINS**	Beans Tofu Red meat Pork Sardines Oysters / Shellfish Lamb meat
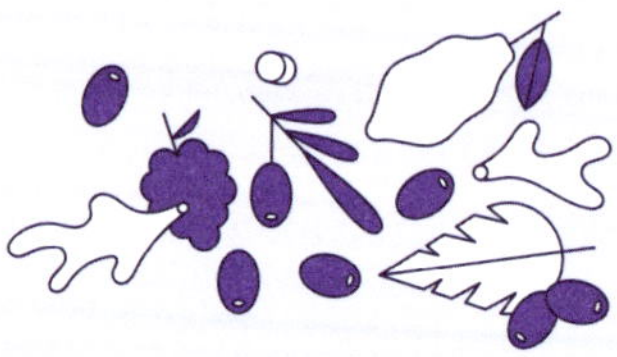	**EXTRAS**	Sea salt Miso Coconut water Bone broth Turmeric Ricotta

FOLLICULAR PHASE (SPRING)	OVULATION PHASE (SUMMER)	PREMENSTRUAL PHASE (AUTUMN)
Asparagus Broccoli Carrots Peas Zucchini Artichokes Edamame Leafy greens Avocados	Arugula Red bell pepper Cucumber Eggplant Endive Fennel Spinach Tomatoes	Pumpkin Sweet potato Parsnip Cauliflower Sprouts Celery Watercress
Oats Quinoa	Quinoa Wholegrain couscous Corn	Brown rice Wild rice Whole grain (spelt) pasta
Cashew nuts Flax seed Brazil nuts Pumpkin seeds	Almonds Pecan nuts Pistachio nuts Sesame seeds Sunflower seeds	Sesame seeds Sunflower seeds Walnuts Hemp seed Chia seeds
Grapefruit Mandarins Cherries Orange Lemon / Lime Plums Pomegranate	Raspberries Strawberries Melon Passion fruit Papaya Pineapple Figs Mango	Apples Pears Peaches Bananas Dates Raisins
Lentils Tofu Trout Eggs Chicken	Eggs Lamb meat Chicken Lentils Beans Salmon Tuna Shrimp	Chickpeas Beans Beef Turkey White fish
Yogurt / Kefir Olives Pickles Vinegar Kimchi Kombucha	Chives Turmeric Ginger Rosemary Sage Parmesan	Tahini Ginger Cinnamon Cocoa Mint Coriander Cottage cheese

Nutrition is the most important source of the right vitamins and minerals to balance your hormones. But even if you eat healthy, it is difficult to get enough and the right dose of micronutrients you need to feel good. Supplements can therefore provide added value in supporting your health.

This food chart serves as inspiration to add things to your meals and bring more variety to your dishes. It is not intended that you eat only these ingredients.

What should you pay attention to when buying dietary supplements?
Make sure you know what you are buying and whether you actually need these extra vitamins and minerals. Choose supplements that contain as few fillers as possible and avoid colorants. Buy supplements that contain active and natural ingredients (they are usually a bit more expensive, but not necessarily the most expensive). Active ingredients are better absorbed by the body. If you buy a supplement, check if it has a notification number. Then you know that the composition has been approved by a health authority (the FDA in the US).

EXERCISE AND YOUR CYCLE

Does your menstrual cycle affect your athletic performance? Not much, you would think. But have you ever wondered why you break all records one week and are completely despondent in the gym a week later? It has a lot to do with your menstrual cycle.

Your hormones influence how you feel and also how your body responds to physical exertion. This is because your pain threshold, recovery and endurance are partly controlled by your hormones. But during the different phases of your menstrual cycle, your hormones and energy levels constantly change, so whether you follow a strict workout schedule or not: unfortunately, there is no magical workout routine that works for everyone.

The female body really works differently than a man's A workout routine that is suitable for a man may not necessarily work for a woman. Therefore, whether or not your workout schedule is successful does not depend on your endurance, but on the fact that your body is different than a man's.

Fortunately, we can also use that to our advantage. Dr. Stacy Sims, PhD, expert in female physiology and endurance training, discovered how to adjust your workouts to your cycle in order to get the most out of yourself. If you get to know your cycle well and become aware of the different phases, you will get more out of your sports sessions, whatever your exercise goal may be. Adapting your exercise to your cycle has many benefits.

You can first and foremost manage stress better. If you exercise for too long and too intensely during the premenstrual phase, you produce too much cortisol. When your body needs to produce more cortisol, it 'steals' estrogen and progesterone, causing an imbalance in your hormones. Keep this in mind during your training sessions. It is important to give your body enough time to recover.

During the luteal phase, your metabolism speeds up. This means that calories are burned faster than usual in the week before your period. Your body needs more calories during this period, about one hundred to three hundred extra per day.

In addition, many women experience cravings in the week before their menstruation, in the final phase. This craving arises from a shift in hormone levels, which causes serotonin levels to be lower. This feel-good hormone ensures that you feel satisfied, satiated, confident and balanced. It suppresses negative feelings.

Extra nutrition can help bring your serotonin levels back in balance. Choose sweet, carbohydrate-rich and complete foods such as fruit, sweet potatoes, honey and dates. Not only are they delicious, but this also makes you feel relaxed thanks to the small serotonin boost. Note: insufficient fuel is a form of stress and has a negative impact on your training and health.

For each season, I give you guidance on how to adjust your training schedule.

TRAINING ACCORDING TO YOUR CYCLE

MENSTRUAL PHASE
WINTER

- gentle form of yoga (Yin yoga, Yoga Nidra, Hatha Yoga)
- walking
- stretching
- if enough energy: start strength training

Follicular phase
SPRING

- Vinyasa yoga
- Pilates
- HIIT workouts (high-intensity interval training)
- cardio training
- walking and running
- cycling
- swimming

OVULATORY PHASE
SUMMER

- power yoga
- Pilates
- kickboxing
- CrossFit
- Bootcamp
- dancing

---

premenstrual phase
AUTUMN

- yoga
- Pilates
- walking
- stretching
- swimming

GO WITH THE FLOW

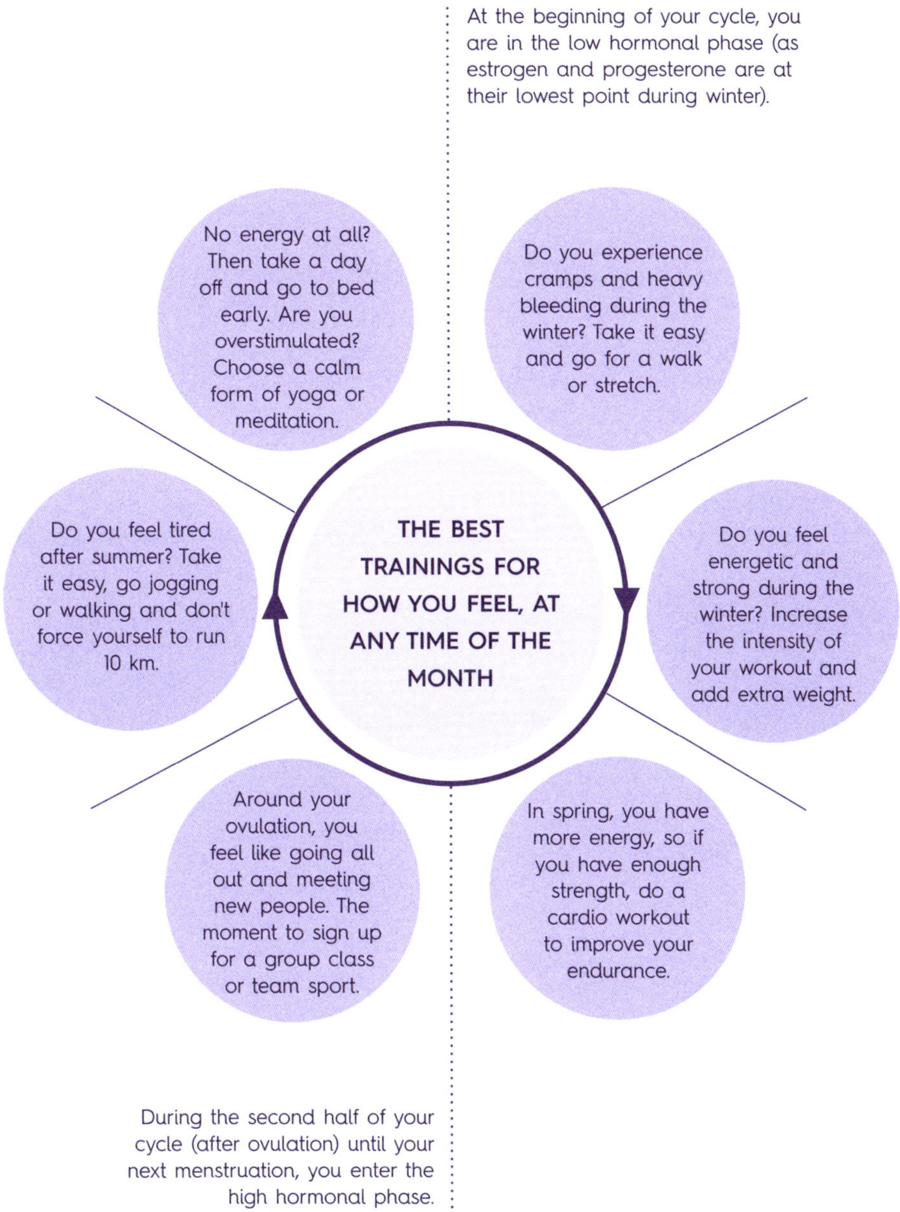

STRESS AND YOUR CYCLE

We all know that stress is not good for our health, but did you know that it can totally confuse your hormones?

We all experience it, stress. There is daily stress, like rushing to be on time for work, and then there is also chronic stress, which can have an impact on your entire body.

We all need stress to function on a daily basis (e.g. the stress of an exam motivates you to study more). But chronic, long-term stress is not so good. Too much stress can take its toll and cause acne, headaches, weight gain, hair loss, mood swings and digestive problems. It can even affect your menstrual cycle and fertility. That is what I have also experienced myself. I didn't realize that I had a lot of internal stress. I always associated stress with work, but I have discovered that your body can also produce more stress when, for example, you exercise too intensely, drink too much coffee or don't sleep well.

Fortunately, your body is smart, because when you experience too much stress, it will put your menstruation and ovulation on hold because it is not ideal to conceive a baby in such a situation. If you don't have a desire to have children, you may not care much about this, but I am convinced that your menstrual health determines your overall health. Even if you don't want children, it's still important to have regular menstrual cycles. And if you have missed periods due to too much stress, then it's time to do something about it.

When your body experiences stress, it produces cortisol. This is the primary stress hormone. To produce more cortisol, your body will steal progesterone, causing your progesterone levels to decrease. And that can disrupt your hormonal balance. It can lead to changes in the frequency and duration of your menstruation and make your menstrual symptoms worse every month.

What causes stress? Not only work or emotional problems can lead to more stress, but also other factors such as intensive workouts, disrupted sleep, too much caffeine, and strict diets.

Stress becomes a problem when you regularly notice one of the following things: your menstruation is late, early, heavier (more blood), more painful, or stops completely (also known as amenorrhea), or you have bleeding between your menstruations.

You need to find a way to relax. That is easier said than done. It also took me a few years to find a routine to reduce or control my stress levels. I was able to tackle the stress thanks to the following seven tips.

1. **Make sleep a priority.** Aim for at least seven hours sleep per night and try to always go to bed at the same time.

2. **Practice mindfulness.** Life can be stressful, but it has been proven that yoga, breathing exercises and meditation help to reduce stress.

3. **Exercise!** Aim for at least 75 minutes of vigorous activity per week and try to move for at least 30 minutes every day. If you are a professional athlete and train every day, you would do well to visit a doctor who specialises in sports medicine. They can give you advice on how to maintain your performance without disrupting your cycle. You should prioritize recovery and rest days at the very least.

4. **Reduce caffeine.** We're not saying you have to give up your morning coffee, but bear in mind that too much caffeine can make you anxious and nervous. Stop drinking coffee for a while or opt for decaffeinated coffee.

5. **Eat plenty of fruit and vegetables and foods that are rich in essential fats** (found in fatty fish such as salmon). These foods help keep your brain healthy and also help balance your hormones.

6. **Increase your magnesium intake.** It has been proven that magnesium calms the nervous system and reduces stress. It can also help you to deal with stress better. You can eat more magnesium-rich foods (green leafy vegetables, dark chocolate, and nuts) or you can choose a supplement with easily absorbable magnesium (such as magnesium citrate and/or bisglycinate).

7. **Have fun!** Do something you enjoy every day. Spend time with friends, laugh, listen to music, dance like nobody's watching. Letting go every now and then can work wonders in reducing cortisol levels.

SLEEP AND YOUR CYCLE

Our sleep, just like our cycle, also occurs in different phases. At night, you go through the same sleep cycle three to six times. Within each cycle, a distinction is made between non-REM sleep and REM sleep. The non-REM sleep consists of four phases: the falling asleep phase, the light sleep phase, the transition phase and the deep sleep phase. The deep sleep phase provides physical rest and recovery. REM sleep, also known as dream sleep, always follows deep sleep and becomes longer and more intense towards the end of the night. After each cycle, there is a very brief moment of awakening, a way for the body to check if everything is still okay. If you receive stimuli at that moment, such as noise or light, you will effectively wake up to solve the problem.

Some 75 to 80 percent of nighttime sleep consists of non-REM sleep, which mainly occurs in the early part of the night.

REM sleep stands for Rapid Eye Movement, because the eyes move continuously during this phase. All muscles in your body are then relaxed. However, your brain and eyes are fully active. If you wake up during your REM sleep, you will feel groggy, tired and disoriented. It is the phase of mental and emotional recovery in which the data stored in long-term memory are processed. If you have had too little REM sleep, you will find it difficult to concentrate the next day.

What do our female hormones have to do with all this? More than you think! There is more and more research showing that changes in estrogen and progesterone hormone levels during the menstrual cycle can affect our sleep quality, both positively and negatively. Progesterone rises after ovulation and plays an active role during the premenstrual phase. That's good news because progesterone is good for sleep. The hormone affects the production of your sleep hormone melatonin and promotes relaxation. In the days before your menstruation, both progesterone and estrogen levels decrease, which can lead to sleep problems. That can cause you to wake up more often at night and have more emotional dreams. That can be frustrating and annoying, and you can feel tired and grumpy during the day.

During the follicular phase (the first part of the menstrual cycle, prior to ovulation), REM sleep lasts longer in many women. That means that our dreams in this phase of our cycle can be more vivid and intense, which offers us a rich source of inspiration and creativity. During our REM sleep, we can actually become sexually aroused, as several studies have found. Almost all men even get an erection multiple times. In women, blood flow increases in the vulva, especially in the clitoris. Sometimes, an intense sexual dream can lead to an orgasm, also in women. Discover more about orgasms on page 140.

Looking for scientifically based sleep advice? Then read the books by neurologist Steven Laureys or by scientist Matthew Walker.

Five tips for better sleep

1. **Establish an evening routine.**
   Unwind with a cup of decaffeinated tea, read a book, take a bath, listen to a sleep meditation, have sex with your partner – whatever helps you relax. Put your phone aside and don't watch TV right before going to bed. The light from those screens can disrupt your melatonin production.

2. **Do not stay in bed awake for more than an hour.**
   If you're lying there staring at the ceiling, then get up and sit in the dark on a chair or sofa. Let go of your thoughts and then, only when you feel sleepy, go back into bed.

3. **Turn your bedroom into an oasis of tranquility.**
   Set your thermostat to a comfortable temperature (cooler is better), keep your pets out of the bedroom, invest in a comfortable mattress and good sheets – prepare yourself for a real good night's sleep.

4. **Avoid coffee in the afternoon.**
   Most people enjoy drinking coffee in the morning to wake up. But in the afternoon or evening, coffee does more harm than good. If you still need that extra energy boost, try a shot of ginger!

5. **Magnesium is your best friend.**
   Studies show that magnesium can help you sleep better because it promotes the production of the sleep hormone melatonin. Add magnesium-rich foods to your diet or take a supplement.

YOUR SKIN AND YOUR CYCLE

During your entire menstrual cycle, your skin changes due to hormonal fluctuations. Depending on which phase you are in your cycle, your skin changes from dry to oily and inflamed. By better understanding your menstrual cycle, you can make better decisions on how to care for your skin and avoid unsettled inflamed skin.

- **Estrogen** provides elasticity and firmness. It also maintains the moisture balance of your skin. A low estrogen level can cause dehydrated skin. Too much estrogen causes estrogen dominance. This can cause skin inflammations. In women whose hormones are produced and processed properly (and who therefore have a well-functioning endocrine system), these changes do not cause many problems. But many women cannot process the extra hormones well. As a result, your skin may be more prone to acne the days before your period.

- **Progesterone** and **testosterone** stimulate sebum production and create a natural oil, a layer that protects the skin. Overproduction causes oily skin and can lead to acne, inflammation and blackheads. After you ovulate, progesterone production increases. The impact of progesterone on the skin can stimulate sebum production and shrink your pores. This together causes clogged pores, which results in pimples. An excess of testosterone causes your skin to produce more oil. This oil is in your pores. When it mixes with bacteria, you can get acne.

- **Cortisol** peaks during periods of stress and can also cause increased sebum production. With chronic stress, your skin becomes more sensitive to conditions such as acne, rosacea and eczema due to this hormone.

YOUR SKINCARE THROUGHOUT YOUR CYCLE

1

DRY AND SENSITIVE

MENSTRUAL PHASE

The hormones estrogen and progesterone are at their lowest, making your skin extra sensitive. During your menstruation, your skin's oil production is low, which can make your skin drier and lack a healthy glow.

Hydrate and nourish your skin sufficiently.

7

CALM

FOLLICULAR PHASE

An increase in estrogen improves moisture balance, making your skin less sensitive. Progesterone levels are still low, so the oil production is not fully activated yet.

Exfoliate your skin, but do not scrub.

14

RADIANT

OVULATION PHASE

At this point in your cycle, estrogen peaks and your skin is at its best: radiant and strong!

Emphasize your glow even more with argan or almond oil.

GREASY

PREMENSTRUAL PHASE

Your skin produces more sebum due to an increase in progesterone. Also, estrogen levels suddenly drop after ovulation, making the skin vulnerable and oily. Due to this condition of your skin, there is a greater chance of pimples.

Cleanse your skin thoroughly both in the morning and in the evening.

28

THE INFLUENCE OF HORMONE DISRUPTORS ON YOUR CYCLE

Every day, your body is exposed to about a hundred chemicals that can be found in your bathroom, kitchen, living room and even in your bed. Some of these chemicals mess with your hormones. They are called hormone disruptors or endocrine disruptors.

Scientific studies link exposure to endocrine disruptors to an increased risk of obesity, lower IQ, reduced fertility, and certain cancers. And as you have already read in this book, hormones play a crucial role in our body.

In your body, these chemicals disrupt the production, transport, binding and breakdown of hormones. This causes your body to function as if it produces more or less hormones than it should. And that is exactly what you don't want. Because your hormones regulate pretty much everything in your body. Your hormones control various important processes: your menstrual cycle, your immune system, your metabolism or appetite, and even your mood.

Hormone disruptors are present almost everywhere. A few examples:

- your plastic container or bottle;
- food such as meat, fish, fruit and vegetables, but also processed food;
- medications;
- in soil (via the groundwater through the residual waste);
- fire retardant substances such as paint, your sofa, cables;
- your beauty products like deodorant, nail polish, (color) shampoo;
- cleaning products.

You cannot say that your shampoo is the direct cause of your migraines, or that your day cream causes PCOS or PMS symptoms. It is usually the combination of different products that exposes you to too many endocrine disruptors.

What can you do to minimize your intake of hormone disruptors?

- Avoid plastic. Use glass instead. Also when heating up your food.
- Wash your vegetables and fruit, vary what you eat. Use cast iron pans.
- Go for natural or eco-friendly cleaning products.
- Choose natural scents (essential oils). Do not use products with perfume. Go for safe brands for your beauty products.
- Wash all your clothing and bedding before using it. Ventilate your house twice a day, and clean regularly.

Keep this rule of thumb in mind: Products that have a strong smell, a beautiful color, or that have a long shelf life contain the most chemical substances.

The most well-known hormone disruptors to avoid
The Netherlands-based foundation Erase all Toxins conducted a study in which 111 popular and well-known personal care products were examined. In 60 percent of these products, one or more endocrine-disrupting substances were found.

Check your bathroom cabinet and inspect your products for these substances:

- Parabens
- Aluminum
- Fluoride
- Benzyl alcohol
- Sodium benzoate
- Phenoxyethanol
- Bisphenol A, S, F (BPA, BPS, BPF)
- Synthetic perfume
- Phthalates
- Mineral oils
- Polyethylene glycol (PEG)
- Sodium Laureth Sulfate (SLS)
- Diethanolamine (DEA)
- Propylene Glycol
- Triclosan
- Dioxins
- Perfluorooctanoic acid (PFOA)

TESTIMONY

Nicole Jardim

(WOMEN'S HEALTH & NUTRITION COACH)

Periods have a bad reputation. And I understand why. Many of us spend weeks out of the month dealing with or anticipating the symptoms that can come with our cycles. Cramps. Moodiness. Bloating. Headaches. Acne.

In our society, all of these things are normalized, alongside the pervasive feelings of shame that often accompany discussions about menstruation. The thing is, our period is not a secret and we should not be resigned to suffering in silence every month. On the contrary, our menstrual cycle is a vital sign of health and its significance should be shouted from the rooftops.

For years now, I have leaned into my cyclical nature, but it wasn't always this way. In my teens and early twenties, my cycle was pure chaos – irregular periods, cramps that would make me see stars, very heavy bleeding and a rollercoaster of emotions. Yep, I certainly know a thing or two about the ups and downs of our hormones!

And then I went on the pill, which initially felt like a miracle. The cramps and heavy periods were gone! I didn't know it then, but the pill was only a temporary fix that masked what was actually a raging hormone imbalance – while also creating a whole new set of symptoms. So, while my period experience was easier, I found myself battling chronic yeast infections, UTIs, hair loss, skin issues and just a general feeling of being unwell at a time in my life when I should have been feeling my best! I tried all the western medical resources, but the doctors I saw had no idea what was wrong with me. All of my tests came back "normal." I spent thousands of dollars on tests and procedures and got... nothing. No answers, and no relief.

After years of dealing with these mystery ailments, I decided I needed to make a change. A friend suggested I see an acupuncturist and with nothing to lose I booked an appointment. During the first session, he gave me more answers than any doctor had given me in years. I knew then and there that I was on the right path. If only I had encountered a holistic practitioner to help me when I was 17, it likely would have changed the trajectory of my life. As it was, it took me a couple of years to get my health back on track. During that time, I changed the way I ate and exercised, got rid of my toxic cleaning and personal care products, worked on my mindset and stress, and tried a variety of integrated healing techniques.

When Morgane and I met each other in New York during the premiere of the Business of Birth Control in 2022 (this documentary is a must-watch, by the way), it was clear we shared a passion for menstrual health and empowering women through knowledge to unlock the power of their cycle. I passionately believe that everyone can (and should) be active participants in their health. And the first step is changing how you eat, because your diet has a huge impact on how you feel every day of the month. Nourishing, nutrient-dense foods can dramatically alter your period experience for the better.

CHAPTER 4

The four seasons of your cycle

CHAPTER 4

The four seasons of your cycle

The natural menstrual cycle starts on the first day of menstruation. We like to compare this period in which you lose blood to winter. The reason why I start this book with autumn (the weeks before your menstrual period) is because most women experience complaints during this luteal phase. Sometimes the complaints are so severe that they affect our daily lives. But meanwhile, we still think we should keep going, are the only ones who feel this way, or quietly suffer.

With Guud Woman, we conducted an external survey in May 2022 among 1,000 Flemish and Dutch women. The results are shocking. I will summarize the most important facts for you.

- Some 90 percent of women experience complaints about their menstruation.

- Women most commonly experience cramps (66 percent), headaches (52 percent), fatigue (50 percent), back pain (49 percent) and mood swings (45 percent).

- Two out of three women believe that this is part of being a woman.

- And that doesn't come from nowhere: Some 31 percent are told by their doctor that the symptoms are just part of being a woman and they have to learn to live with them.

- More than a quarter of women do not know who to turn to with their problems.

UNDERSTANDING YOUR MENSTRUAL CYCLE

The length of a regular cycle varies between 22 and 40 days.
The first day of your cycle is the first day of your bleeding.

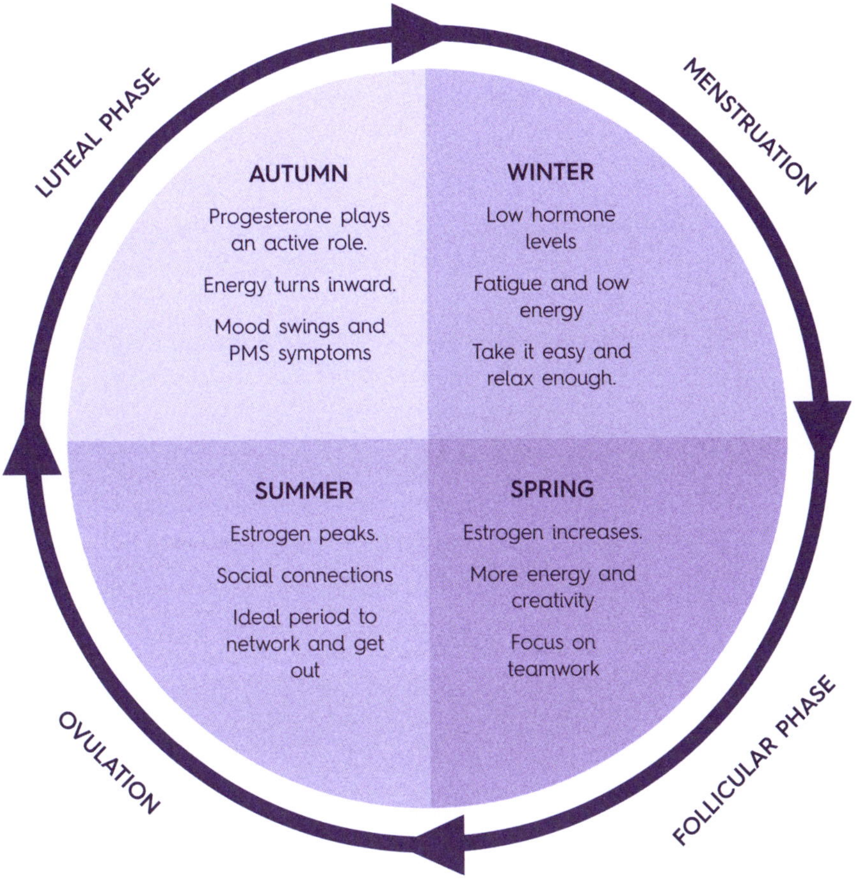

AUTUMN

AUTUMN

Autumn is the ideal time to let go, withdraw and prepare for winter. For many women, autumn is synonymous with the 'PMS season'. Time to take it easy. And believe me, it doesn't make sense to keep performing and functioning the way you do during the other seasons of your cycle. Take time for yourself, be kind to your body, to make it easier for yourself when you experience certain complaints. In autumn, I tend to be stricter and more critical of the people around me, but especially of myself. When I didn't live according to my cycle, I used to have a lot of trouble with severe mood swings in this phase. The little voice inside me brought me down: I wasn't good enough, not loved enough, not beautiful enough, not smart enough, not exciting enough. These were always very difficult days to get through, but since discovering the power of my cycle, I can place these feelings much better and have learned to break these patterns. I now enjoy listening to my body and taking it easy. I have also learned to ask for help more during this period of my cycle, so I don't feel like I am on my own. Saying no more often to social activities also helps to pay more attention to what I really need to support my body.

Phase: the luteal (premenstrual) phase
Duration*: 10 to 14 *days

What is it? The luteal phase is the time after your ovulation and before your menstruation. After ovulation, the remnants of the follicle transform into a yellow body, the corpus luteum, hence the name 'luteal phase'. This yellow body produces progesterone in addition to estrogen. The uterine lining prepares for possible implantation. The cervical mucus becomes sticky again and decreases in quantity. If you measure your basal body temperature, you will also notice that it rises by a few tenths of a degree around or after ovulation and remains elevated until the end of your cycle. The increased temperature indicates that ovulation has occurred and that the fertile period is over.

If you have had sex during your ovulation and your egg is fertilized, your body produces gonadotropin (hCG), the hormone that can be detected by a pregnancy test. Your progesterone level continues to rise to maintain pregnancy, which is why progesterone is called the 'pregnancy hormone.' If you have been pregnant before, you may remember that you were very tired during the first few weeks. That is due to the increase in progesterone.

If your egg is not fertilized during ovulation, the yellow body dies and there is a sudden drop in estrogen and progesterone. Your basal body temperature will also start to decrease again. The mucous membrane is shed during menstruation, about twelve to sixteen days after ovulation. This is the beginning of your menstruation and the start of a new cycle.

HOW DOES THE MENSTRUAL CYCLE PROCEED?

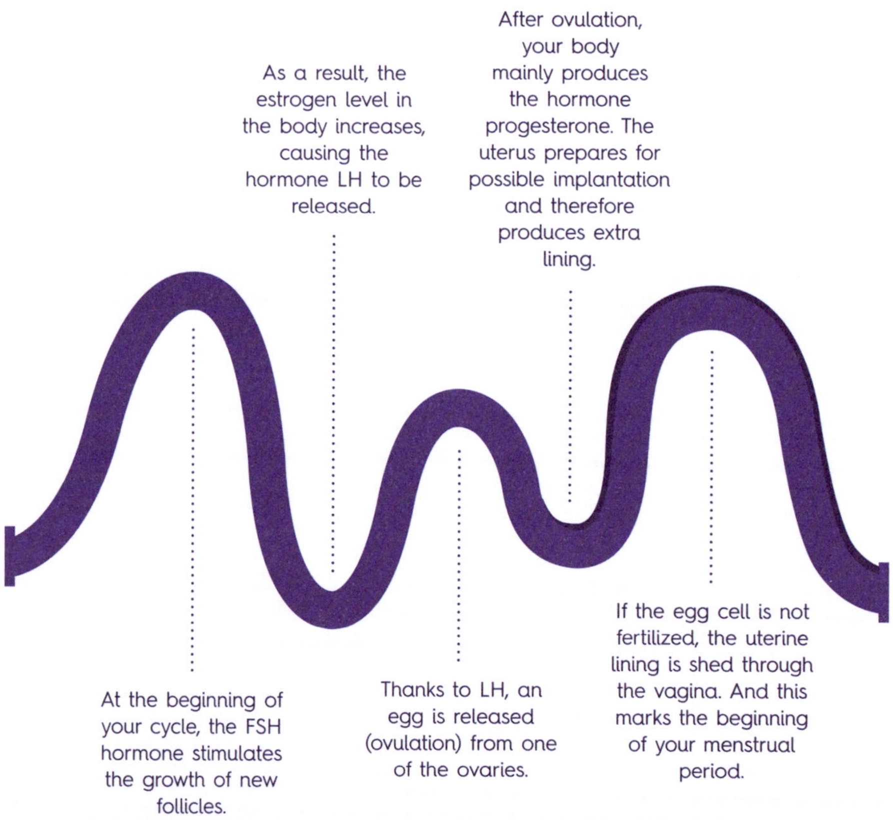

Difficult to get pregnant? Maybe your luteal phase is too short.

Rebecca Verhofstede, midwife and Sensiplan coach, explains: Did you know that a normal luteal phase lasts between ten and sixteen days? The luteal phase is considered short if it lasts less than ten days. A deficiency of progesterone during the second half of your cycle can cause the luteal phase to be shortened. But with a deficiency of progesterone, the duration of this phase can also be normal. If the luteal phase is too short or if there is insufficient production of progesterone (<10 μg/L mid-luteal), we refer to luteal insufficiency.

A shortage of progesterone can cause your uterine lining to be broken down too quickly, preventing a fertilized egg from having enough time to properly implant in the uterus. It can be a cause of reduced fertility and therefore more difficulty in getting pregnant, but also of an early miscarriage.

HOW YOU FEEL DURING AUTUMN

Why is this phase called autumn? In autumn, the weather is stormy, just like your hormones in this phase. Due to the rapid decrease in the hormones estrogen and progesterone just before menstruation, many women experience PMS symptoms such as cramps, headaches, acne, bloating and mood swings. And just like trees prepare for a cold winter by shedding their leaves, you feel your energy turning inward. It is a preparation for winter, where you turn even further within yourself. At the end of this phase, your energy level decreases and you feel tired, both physically and mentally.

You might feel a bit down in autumn. Therefore, in this phase you focus on:

- Self-care. Take care of your body with a soothing massage or enjoy an extra long bath with a delicious herbal tea.
- Take on easy tasks that don't require much mental exertion and don't be too critical of yourself. Talk to yourself like you would to your best friend, because you are so worth it!
- Feel like staying indoors? Then definitely do it. Maybe an evening on the couch with a good movie is exactly what you need.

- Keep moving, but take it easy. Go for a walk in the countryside, do some stretching or a gentle form of yoga to feel better.

In the days before your menstruation, you often notice an emotional change due to the hormones estrogen and progesterone. As you already know by now, your hormones rise and fall throughout your entire cycle. The sudden drop in estrogen just after ovulation and just before menstruation can affect neurotransmitters or 'messenger molecules' in your brain, such as serotonin and dopamine. These are both so-called 'happiness hormones' that influence your well-being, your mood, your sleep and your energy level. In this phase, you assess yourself, are critical and may experience intense mood swings.

Once your menstruation starts, the hormone levels stabilize again and your mood should improve.

If PMS or PMDD seriously affects your daily life, contact your doctor for help. You don't have to suffer.

What is PMDD?

Premenstrual dysphoric disorder (PMDD) is a cyclic, hormone-based mood disorder. During the premenstrual phase, certain symptoms occur (panic attacks, extreme mood swings, feelings of despair, and severe depressive symptoms). It is estimated that this condition occurs in 5 to 8 percent of women during their reproductive years. PMDD is a severe negative reaction to the natural rise and fall of estrogen and progesterone. It is believed to be a disorder at the cellular level, with symptoms that worsen over time as well as sometimes during menstruation, pregnancy, childbirth, miscarriage and perimenopause.

DO ALL WOMEN REALLY HAVE TO DEAL WITH PMS DURING THEIR AUTUMN?

PMS stands for premenstrual syndrome and is a collective term for severe physical complaints that you can experience in the period before your menstruation. Research shows that nine out of ten women suffer from menstrual complaints. Half of them take painkillers monthly to alleviate these complaints.

The main characteristic of PMS is that the complaints are related to your menstrual cycle. They are so severe that they really dominate the days around your menstruation. Think of mood swings, fatigue, low energy, irritability, cramps, headaches, migraines, bloating, water retention, unsettled skin or painful and tight breasts. Do you experience these complaints and do they restrict what you can do during the day? Then it is best to visit a doctor.

It is not entirely clear how some women can have many complaints and others can go through their menstruation almost unscathed. Doctors believe that women with PMS are more sensitive to hormonal fluctuations. It also appears that women with PMS often have too much estrogen. This is called estrogen dominance. Although the exact cause is not entirely clear, chronic stress, lack of self-care, unhealthy diet, environmental factors, and hormone disruptors could potentially have an impact on your hormonal balance and contribute to estrogen dominance.

A blood test can be useful when you have a hormonal imbalance. In this way, you can get a better understanding of your hormone levels and gain more information about your health. You can detect fertility problems, and find out which phase of your menstrual cycle you are in and whether you are in perimenopause. You should discuss with your doctor or hormonal coach at what moment it is best to have a test done, because the results can vary depending on the phase of your cycle.

HOW TO ALLEVIATE YOUR PMS SYMPTOMS

What works for one person doesn't always work for the other. See for yourself what makes a difference for you, but bear in mind that change takes time. Give yourself three months to feel the effect if you make any changes to your lifestyle.

1. **Take a close look at your diet**
   If you have too much estrogen, it is important that your body can break it down and excrete it properly. You do this by eating the right foods. Good nutrients help to break down the excess estrogen better. Think about the right fatty acids, leafy greens, and fibers. Also, avoid coffee, sugar and alcohol, certainly during the premenstrual phase.

2. **Reduce stress**
   Studies have revealed that stress can worsen PMS symptoms. This is tricky, as it is of course a vicious circle: you don't feel well and that causes stress. But because of that stress, you feel even worse. However, it is a good idea to take a moment to think about it. Maybe there is a way to reduce your stress. Reduce your workload for a while, be kind to yourself, decide whether or not to make certain appointments, or simply treat yourself to a nice relaxing evening.

Tip

Have you tried meditation? If you don't have any experience with this yet, it can sometimes feel intimidating to start. But that is really not necessary. There are useful apps that help you disconnect for 10 minutes a day and focus on your breathing to find peace again. You don't have to meditate in silence for hours to notice a positive difference in your stress levels. Be sure to check out the Calm app.

3. **Exercise, but not too much**
   If you suffer from PMS complaints, you often don't feel much like exercising. However, physical activity can help to alleviate your symptoms. So get off the couch and unroll your yoga mat, or go for a brisk walk. When you exercise, endorphins (happiness hormones) are also released. You feel better and have more energy. Note: if you exercise too intensively during your premenstrual phase, you can exacerbate certain symptoms. Listen to your body carefully and don't force yourself to run ten kilometers if you don't feel up to it. During the premenstrual phase, your body needs more time to recover, so keep this in mind.

4. **Sleep better, not more**
   Good sleep is necessary for your physical and mental well-being. How many hours of sleep you need depends on the person, but most people need at least seven hours of sleep to feel good. Sleep is important so that your body can recover.

YOUR WORK/LIFE DURING AUTUMN: A PHASE OF FINISHING AND CLEANING UP

Your behavior can be difficult to predict during this period. It is a phase in which you may feel that you have less energy. It is the ideal time to finish projects. You may feel that you are more critical (of yourself and others), which allows you to examine things in more detail. Complete projects, perform administrative tasks such as bookkeeping, tidy up your desk, and hand in your monthly reports.

YOUR SLEEP DURING AUTUMN

A lower sleep quality during the premenstrual phase and during menstruation is common in women with premenstrual symptoms or painful menstrual cramps. These can be explained by estrogen dominance. That means you have too much estrogen in relation to progesterone. This can cause PMS symptoms and therefore also decreased sleep quality. Estrogen dominance is caused by a combination of many different factors, including stress, lack of self-care, poor nutrition, a sedentary lifestyle and exposure to environmental toxins.

At the beginning of the premenstrual phase (the days after your ovulation), women often have more non-REM sleep, which is associated with a deeper, more restful sleep. In the morning, you feel fresher, better rested and ready to start the day.

Two to three days before your menstruation, you will experience a sudden drop in estrogen and progesterone levels. During this time, many women experience sleep problems. You may notice that you wake up more often at night and your dreams become more emotional. During these days, for example, I suffer more from hot flashes and my pajamas are sometimes soaking wet. I know then that my period will come a few days later. Of course, not every woman experiences these changes in the same way. Some women do not notice any difference in their sleep quality during their menstrual cycle, while others notice that their sleep is affected by the phase they are in. Most problems start after ovulation, when cortisol levels rise. Your body temperature is therefore slightly higher. Around 12 to 24 hours after ovulation, your body temperature rises (due to the hormone progesterone) by about 0.3 to 0.5 degrees Celsius or 0.5 to 0.9 degrees of Fahrenheit. Sometimes the temperature rise occurs a bit later. Your temperature remains high and drops just before the next menstruation to the level of the first day of the cycle.

BASAL BODY TEMPERATURE DURING YOUR CYCLE.

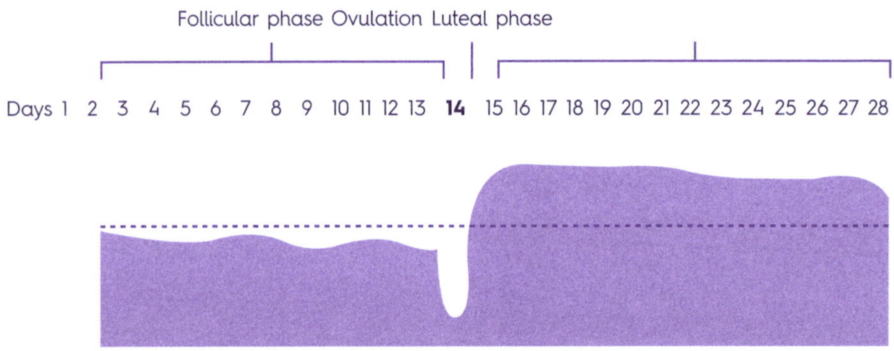

Research shows that the intensity of your dreams can also depend on your body temperature. The temperature of a woman rises around ovulation and suddenly drops again when she gets her period. This change in temperature is due to hormonal fluctuations in your cycle and can lead to vivid dreams.

If you experience sleep problems, I recommend keeping a sleep diary. This way, you can identify patterns and take action to improve your sleep quality and feel better during the day.

YOUR DIET DURING AUTUMN

Progesterone plays an active role during the premenstrual phase. So choose foods that are rich in zinc (shellfish such as oysters and mussels, fish, nuts), magnesium (green leafy vegetables, bananas, seeds, meat), vitamin C (citrus fruits, kiwi, bell peppers, tomatoes), and vitamin B6 (lentils, chickpeas, cruciferous vegetables, seeds) to support this hormone.

Furthermore, it is important to keep your blood sugar levels stable (see p. 58), because progesterone can cause a significant drop. Avoid spikes and dips in your blood sugar levels by adding complex carbohydrates and fiber-rich foods. Choose whole grain products and lots of vegetables. I, for example, like to eat beets during this period because it can help regulate your blood sugar levels. Do not start your day with fruit juice and granola, but opt for a savory breakfast like an egg with avocado and a slice of whole wheat bread. If you start the day with too much sugar or glucose (also called blood sugar), you soon feel tired and hungry.

If you eat complex carbohydrates, your blood sugar will rise slowly and so your body will also not produce insulin too quickly or too much. When your blood sugar reaches its peak, it also slowly drops again. When you choose fast carbs, your blood sugar rises very quickly, causing your body to produce a lot, usually too much, insulin. After the peak, your blood sugar level will then drop very quickly, resulting in energy dips. Your energy quickly starts looking for new energy and you reach for sugar again. You end up in a vicious cycle, where you constantly want sugar and experience cravings or binge eating.

If you want to learn more about how to keep your blood sugar levels stable, prepare to be inspired by the book Glucose Revolution by Jessie Inchauspé. Since I started following her on Instagram (@glucosegoddess), I have learned that it's not what I eat that is important, but rather the order in which I eat that has a big impact on my mood, energy levels and menstrual health.

I have never been a fan of diets, especially not counting calories, but what I do want to mention here is that your body needs more calories, between 100 and 300 extra, during autumn. This is not an excuse to eat an extra slice of pizza or a bag of crisps, but do make sure you eat enough. Add complex carbohydrates (sweet potato, wild rice, whole wheat pasta) and proteins (poultry, eggs, legumes, beans, nuts) for a satisfied feeling after your meals. If you don't get enough protein from your diet, it can be a good idea to add plant-based protein powder to your smoothie or yogurt, or eat a protein bar as a snack.

How much protein do you need? Proteins are the building blocks of your body. It is important that you have enough of it, not just for a satisfied feeling. They allow your body to recover properly and keep your muscles strong.

As you get older, proteins also play an important role in protecting your bones. From my own experience, I know that it is difficult to get enough protein each day. The recommended amount for a woman is 0.8 grams per kilogram of body weight. In my case, that would be 0.8 x 58 kg = 46 grams of protein per day. If you do strength training and want to gain more muscle mass, you need more proteins, namely between 1.6 and 2.2 grams per kilogram of body weight.

Avoid alcohol, coffee, black tea, processed food, white carbohydrates, refined sugar, gluten and dairy. I have personally experienced that they only amplify your complaints. Moreover, they cause more inflammation in your body, and due to the sudden drop in estrogen and progesterone just before your period, your body is already more sensitive to this. Add herbs to your diet that have anti-inflammatory properties.

The power of herbs

Herbs can provide incredible support to your body during your cycle. They can be used to balance both estrogen and progesterone, improve hormone processing, replenish missing minerals and vitamins, and fight inflammation. Each herb provides its own unique medicinal powers, but **nutrition expert and herbalist Lily Joan Roberts** has singled out a few that can make a world of difference for many women during autumn.

- Chamomile: anti-inflammatory, improves digestion, relaxes muscles and the nervous system, and reduces menstrual cramps.

- Ginger: anti-inflammatory, antispasmodic and promotes blood circulation in the uterus, helping you get rid of your cramps faster.

- Fennel: reduces tension and spasms and helps with bloating or digestive problems that sometimes occur during PMS.

- **Dandelion:** supports your liver in detoxification, helps with digestive problems, and reduces inflammation.

- **Raspberry leaf:** helps strengthen and relax your uterine muscles, and has a soothing effect on menstrual cramps and other autumn complaints.

The best way to take these herbs is in the form of tea. Mix the herbs in equal amounts, for example two tablespoons per herb. If you use ginger, it is best to use dried pieces. Shake and store this mixture in a sealed jar.

To make an infusion, take two tablespoons of the mix and pour 500 milliliters of boiling water over it. Let it steep for 15 minutes. A tip: a *French press* is very handy for this, then you can push the spices through. Drink this tea throughout the day.

If you suffer badly from PMS symptoms, you can also add cramp bark (aslo known as Guelder rose). Other more special herbs that are known for their healing properties include schisandra, black cohosh, evening primrose oil and St. John's wort.

Alcohol during your menstrual cycle

Your menstrual cycle could have an impact on your hangovers. Maybe you notice that sometimes you drink a lot and still wake up fine, while other times you have a hangover from just one drink. What is going on?

Women may be more sensitive to the effects of alcohol the week before their menstruation. The reason? Estrogen. After ovulation, the liver has to break down estrogen. If you drink a lot of alcohol during these days, the combination of alcohol and estrogen can put a strain on the liver and cause problems such as headaches, water retention and bloating.

Try to avoid alcohol during the premenstrual phase; it only exacerbates your menstrual symptoms.

Have you had one too many?

- **Drink a lot.**
  And, of course, I don't mean alcohol or coffee. The caffeine in coffee will dehydrate you even more. Try to drink a lot of water!

- **Sleep in and have some sex.**
  Not too bad, right?! During sleep, your body recovers faster, and when you have sex, your body produces the hormone oxytocin, which reduces pain stimuli and makes you feel good. Self-pleasure counts too!

- **Eat something.**
  Try to start the day with a healthy breakfast, even if all you feel like is chocolate croissants. Whole grain bread and fruit are healthy and safe options, but an egg and avocado are of course the ultimate hangover food as a source of proteins, vitamin B and healthy fats. Drink ginger tea or green tea to detoxify your body.

- **Exercise outdoors.**
  Exercise helps your body break down alcohol more easily. And fresh air is always good for you.

YOUR SKIN DURING AUTUMN

Your skin during autumn can sometimes feel a bit unsettled. Due to an increase in progesterone, you may produce more sebum, resulting in pimples. This period is therefore the moment to take good care of your skin with soothing, natural products.

Tip

You can also take care of your skin from the inside out. Choose foods rich in zinc, vitamin A (in the form of beta-carotene), selenium and vitamin C to support your skin. If you cannot obtain these vitamins and minerals from your diet, remember to add a high-quality supplement.

Skincare advice from Marion Naudts (Marion Maakt), expert in skincare.

With her books and workshops, she has already inspired many women to make their own natural care products. Now she has also developed a special line that is tailored to the different phases of the cycle. I'm already a fan and wanted to find out what her personal care routine looks like.

'During my cycle, I don't change my basic skincare routine: my favorite gentle cleanser, a hydrating tonic, and my moisturizer as a day and night cream. What I do, however, is add extras according to the needs of my skin in the different phases.

Progesterone plays an active role in autumn and activates sebum production. Excessive sebum clogs your pores and forms the ideal breeding ground for bacteria that cause pimples. It is important to cleanse your skin well in the morning and evening.

Due to the increase in progesterone, your pores become clogged more quickly and your skin becomes oilier. These are ideal conditions for bacteria that cause acne. In this phase of my cycle, I like to use skincare products that keep the pores open and target the acne bacteria. Salicylic acid is a commonly used ingredient for this. That has an exfoliating and therefore intestinal cleansing effect. I am not a fan of synthetic salicylic acid, but prefer to use the plant-based alternative from, for example, willow or wintergreen. Again, it is important to be kind to your skin and not try to tackle pimples with the big guns. This does not pay off in the long run.

Do you experience persistent pimples at any time during your cycle? In that case, I would advise against exfoliating your skin with acids in the initial stage. First and foremost, focus on restoring your skin barrier. This can be done by using a mild cleanser and cream, supplemented by, say, the same serum you would use during your menstruation.'

What about hormonal acne?

If you suffer from (hormonal) acne, that is actually a cry for help from your body. Hormonal acne is a problem that many women experience, even if their teenage years are long gone.

Acne is caused by clogged pores on your face. Ordinary pimples sometimes occur due to makeup or sweat that accumulates in your pores. Hormonal acne occurs when hormonal changes in your body cause your skin to produce more oil or trigger inflammation. Women experience hormonal fluctuations throughout the entire month. Why do some people get acne while others have clear skin? Some women do not efficiently process the excess estrogen, progesterone and testosterone that your body produces throughout the month. If your body doesn't deal with these hormones properly, it can cause acne. If your cycle is natural and functioning well, these hormonal changes don't make much of a difference. But if you are one of the unlucky ones who cannot handle the hormones correctly, you may suffer from acne every month. No matter how tempting it may be, do not squeeze your pimples; leave them alone. The chances are high that you will otherwise get scars that will probably never disappear. I know it's difficult, but really don't do it. Pimples disappear, scars don't. Many doctors and people around you may recommend hormonal contraception or antibiotics. It can work, but the long-term side effects should not be ignored.

What can you do against acne?

1. Pay attention to your diet and lifestyle. Coffee, chemicals, lack of sleep, the pill and stress strip your body of important nutrients that keep your hormones healthy and ensure clear skin.
2. Excessive alcohol consumption and sugar intake cause the liver to work overtime. Your liver needs sufficient nutrients to detoxify your body. If it is too busy getting rid of things like alcohol and sugar, it won't be able to get rid of your excess estrogen. This results in estrogen dominance, which in turn causes pimples.
3. During the second half of your cycle (after ovulation until your period), your progesterone level will rise. Progesterone causes increased sebum production, resulting in pimples. A zinc supplement can then work supportively for your skin.
4. Take care of your gut health. An imbalanced gut flora is also linked to acne. On page 60, I will tell you more about it.

Sometimes, the hardest thing to wear is our own skin. But remember even with scars, pimples and wounds you are beautiful. Free yourself from judgement and shame, as you vibrate higher daily.

UNKNOWN

YOUR SEX DRIVE DURING AUTUMN

After ovulation, you may experience a slight dip due to a decrease in estrogen. But just because you're in your autumn doesn't mean you can't experience delightful arousals. You may feel less horny and attractive than during your summer. But it's important that you learn to listen to your body and open yourself up to getting to know and embrace your sexuality in different ways and at different times.

That means for me: knowing what I like (thanks to self-pleasure) and what I don't enjoy as much. That also includes learning to enjoy and receive, setting my boundaries and being able to say no, so that I can say yes wholeheartedly. During this phase of my cycle, I always feel a bit less loved and I am more critical of myself and the people around me. Now that I am aware of this, I prioritize self-care and self-pleasure in this phase, and I try to let go of control and reconnect with myself. I take a warm bath, let myself be massaged with oil or take the time to enjoy a wonderful orgasm when I masturbate. If you don't feel like masturbating, then simply stroking or touching yourself can also work wonders to reconnect with yourself.

Tip

Do you feel like you love yourself less during the week before your period? Stand in front of the mirror naked every day and say out loud what you find beautiful about yourself. After giving birth and breastfeeding, I struggled to look at my body. My breasts were no longer as firm as before and everything looked a bit different. I felt less attractive because of it, and that also had an impact on my sex life. For three months, I stood naked in front of the mirror every day and said out loud what I liked about my body and what I was grateful for. This exercise was very powerful for me. I felt better about myself and was proud of my breasts again, which ultimately allowed me to breastfeed my son for nine weeks. Fantastic, right?

EXERCISE DURING AUTUMN

This phase is about mobility and recovery. It is fine if you feel you don't have much energy and can only do less than usual. Research shows that women during their autumn become tired more quickly and need more time to recover. Choose gentle and slow activities, and light weights. Focus on flexibility and technique and work on your posture.

Don't force yourself to run ten kilometers, replace intense workouts with a gentle form of yoga or Pilates. In this phase where I don't exercise much, I go on long evening walks to relax.

Tip

If you still have plenty of energy, then I am the last person to stop you from going all out, but make sure you have nutritious meals and a good night's sleep so that your body can recover properly.

TESTIMONY

Eva Daeleman

(WRITER, COACH)

"How I plan my life according to the four seasons"

For years, I had the feeling of not really knowing myself. I was living on autopilot and as I was used to. Or rather, as was expected of me. Since I discovered the four seasons of my cycle, I live again through my feminine power. By following the seasons, I feel closer to myself, both physically and mentally. For instance, during the days after my period, in spring, I have more energy and feel like planning social activities and exercising. I take better care of myself now during the autumn, in the days leading up to my period.

When we look outside, we are actually constantly guided by the seasons. Our technological developments have brought us many comforts, but unfortunately we are also increasingly distant from nature. It has meant so much to me to take the seasons into account. And to listen more to my body. It has taken the sharp edges off, I have become much less strict with myself and am gentler with my body. The seasons support me: in my autumn, I make sure I have warming comfort food, do gentle exercise and allow myself those naps I crave so much. In winter, I wear comfortable clothes, keep my schedule free from extra appointments, and can therefore go to bed nice and early. During my summer and spring, I try to make the most of this time by going out as much as possible, picking up my exercise routine and choosing bolder clothes. It feels so natural to follow those waves and not always try to peak.

“It has meant so much to me to take the seasons into account. And to listen more to my body.”

EVA DAELEMAN

WINTER

WINTER

Winter is not my favorite season of the year. I don't really like dark and cold days, but I do like winter during my cycle. The reason for that is that I am always very happy when I get my period. Many women experience bleeding as something dirty and unpleasant, but when I menstruate, I feel so relieved. It also feels like a new beginning, because the first day of your menstruation is also the first day of your cycle. If you have an irregular cycle due to PCOS, like me, I can assure you that you always do a dance of joy when you get your period. A tip that I often give to women is: celebrate your periods. Even though you have a desire to have children and may be disappointed, the fact that you, as a woman, menstruate means that your system is working. A new opportunity to fertilize your egg during your next ovulation.

Phase: the menstrual phase
Duration: 3 to 7 days

Your menstrual cycle starts on the first day of your menstruation. Your estrogen and progesterone levels are at their lowest. Once your body receives the signal that your egg is not fertilized (and therefore no implantation will occur), the progesterone level decreases. This causes the uterine lining to dissolve and your period to start.

Why is this phase called winter? Just like in winter, during this phase you probably have less energy and get tired more quickly. There is no growth; it is rather a time of shedding and letting go. The menstrual phase is therefore a period of rest and reflection.

Also, as in autumn, don't hesitate to put your social calendar on hold. You will be amazed at how much of a difference that makes. There is nothing wrong with living according to the rhythm of your body and listening to your feelings. I personally hate it when I have to pretend to be happy and carefree with friends or acquaintances at times when I'm actually feeling a bit emotional and slightly irritated. With my real friends, I can be 100 percent myself and honestly say that I really don't feel like meeting up but would like to see them later.

Fortunately, winter is not forever. You might suffer from cramps during the days you bleed, and feel tired, irritable and cranky. The more the days pass, the better you feel. Your estrogen level increases, you feel sharper and you have better focus.

HORMONAL FLUCTUATIONS DURING YOUR CYCLE

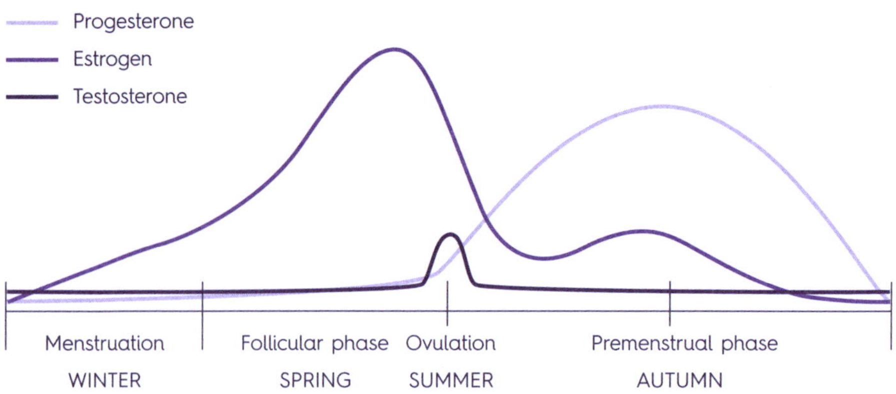

The days after your period, you will notice that you have more energy and that your mood is better. One reason could be that estrogen is linked to serotonin, a neurotransmitter that plays a role in your moods. As estrogen levels increase, serotonin production also increases, which can lead to feelings of happiness and well-being.

Important during your menstruation:

- Do not push yourself too hard during the first days of your menstruation.
- Rest when you are tired. Get enough sleep.
- Choose nutritious meals when you're hungry.
- Take it easy with exercising. Go for a walk, do some yoga, or do some light stretching exercises.
- Don't feel like being surrounded by a lot of people? Just say no, that's okay.

YOUR WORK/LIFE DURING WINTER: A NEW BEGINNING, A PHASE OF REFLECTION AND LETTING GO

Yes, it's that time of the month!You probably don't feel your best during your menstruation. It is a good time to focus on tasks that do not require much social contact and that you can do calmly on your own. Look back on the past weeks and see how you can prepare for the upcoming weeks. Get ready for more productive days, organize your work and tidy up. Try to take it easy and make sure to set aside enough time to relax and let go, you deserve it.

YOUR SLEEP DURING WINTER

Just a few days before the start of your menstruation, your estrogen and progesterone levels decrease. Many women struggle with sleeping. You may also experience more nightmares. Dinteruring your menstruation, you may feel even sleepier than usual; that's because you're losing blood. Therefore, it is important to get enough iron, magnesium and zinc. Try to go to bed around the same time every evening, and aim to get seven to eight hours of sleep.

What is premenstrual syndrome?

Many women suffer from PMS (premenstrual syndrome) because the hormones estrogen and progesterone suddenly drop in the days before menstruation. Some women also experience symptoms in the days after their menstruation. This is called premenstrual syndrome. The symptoms can vary from physical symptoms, such as headaches, to emotional symptoms, such as anxiety.

During your menstruation or the first few days after your menstruation, estrogen levels are still very low. Estrogen is also known as the feel-good hormone. It creates a positive feeling and helps you better cope with stress. In addition, it helps your brain to produce serotonin, endorphins and dopamine, everything you need to feel good. The higher your estrogen level rises, the more mood-enhancing neurotransmitters your brain produces. In the days after your menstruation the estrogen level can still be low, which can make you feel less good about yourself. You can treat postmenstrual complaints in the same way as premenstrual complaints. Try to keep your daily stress under control, make sure you get enough sleep and exercise regularly. Add foods rich in phytoestrogens to your meals. Phytoestrogen is a plant-based estrogen that can be found in foods such as edamame, flaxseed, miso paste, tofu, black beans, sesame seeds, broccoli and kale. Phytoestrogens can mimic the effects of estrogen in case of a deficiency. That is nice during the days after your menstruation, when your estrogen levels are low. These phytoestrogens are also a good idea for menopausal women, as they also produce much less oestrogen.

YOUR DIET DURING WINTER

During winter, you tend to seek warmth. Therefore, choose warm meals such as soups and stews instead. Since you lose blood during this period, it is important to eat enough food rich in iron, zinc and magnesium. I am not a big meat eater myself, but during this phase I do crave red meat. When I go to a restaurant during my winter phase, I often choose steak with fries.

- Make sure you get enough omega-3 throughout your entire cycle. Increase your omega-3 intake with wild salmon, sardines, mackerel, sesame seeds, pumpkin seeds, flax seeds and walnuts.

- Also make sure to get extra magnesium. This powerful mineral can work preventively against cramps and headaches. You can find it in dark leafy greens, nuts, seeds, bananas, raw cacao, fish and shellfish, avocados and supplements.

- Furthermore, you can eat extra iron-rich food during your menstruation. For example, a bouillon from bones and meat made by simmering for hours. Other iron-rich sources include beetroot, watercress, sesame seeds, goji berries, oats, quinoa, buckwheat, dark leafy greens, dates, (dried) apricots, almonds, nettle tea and blackstrap molasses. Iron is actually better absorbed by the body when it is combined with vitamin C. So make sure you have enough citrus fruits, kiwis, strawberries, berries, cabbage, bell peppers, tomatoes, broccoli and sweet potatoes!

YOUR SEX DRIVE DURING WINTER

Winter can make you want to stay in bed, usually because you don't feel well, or have cramps or heavy bleeding. So sex is usually far from your mind, but did you know that orgasms can help with menstrual pain? Worth a try, if you feel like it of course.

What happens when you experience an orgasm? The part of the brain responsible for our thoughts (the prefrontal cortex) becomes inactive. Therefore, we are fearless and less rational during sex. It also produces a juicy cocktail of hormones such as endorphins, dopamine, serotonin and oxytocin. They ensure that an orgasm feels blissful and can act as a natural painkiller to alleviate menstrual discomfort and pain.

Studies have also shown that orgasms can actually help alleviate symptoms of stress. It is important to know that orgasms change in intensity and sensation during your cycle. One week your orgasm can be explosive and the next more subtle. Before blaming your partner, remember that this is completely normal and directly related to how your hormones change during your cycle. If you want to approach it scientifically, try tracking your orgasms throughout the month. Maybe you see a pattern!

YOUR SKIN DURING WINTER

During the menstrual phase, your energy level is often lower and you would rather crawl under a blanket on the couch. Also your skin looks more tired during this period. Not only is it less hydrated, but it also becomes irritated more easily. A low estrogen level during your menstruation causes your skin to feel dry. Use a moisturizing cream, or hydrate from within by drinking plenty of water.

A common mistake people make is to actively tackle pimples during the menstrual phase, for example with peels, intense scrubs ... Just like yourself, your skin simply wants calm and balance.

“

Your menstrual cycle is a key indicator of your overall health – men don’t have this luxury!

UNKNOWN

”

EXERCISE DURING WINTER

Be kind to your body and avoid heavy exertion when exercising. The ideal activity during menstruation varies greatly from woman to woman. If you have enough energy, you can train intensively, because during the first half of your cycle you build muscle more easily. If you still feel too weak, it is important to listen to your body and take it easy. Do not stay in bed or on the couch, because by moving you produce endorphins, which make you feel better and experience less pain.

→ If you don't experience any menstrual symptoms, you can do heavy weight training, because when your estrogen and progesterone hormones are at their lowest, you can recover more easily and train intensively. If you have menstrual complaints, choose a yin yoga session or go for a gentle walk to alleviate your cramps.

The influence of yoga on your menstrual health

I love yoga, and since I completed a yoga teacher training six years ago, I try to unroll my mat every day, even if it's just for 20 minutes, for a good start to the day. It's not just mindful, but it also makes me feel at ease and keeps me flexible. Studies have shown that yoga can have a positive impact on your menstrual health and hormonal balance. Some types of yoga are better suited to the different phases of your cycle. During the first half of your menstrual cycle, it is easier to build muscles because you have more energy. Then choose Vinyasa or power yoga. During the phase before your menstruation, it is better to choose a more gentle yoga session such as yin yoga or Hatha yoga, because your body needs more rest.

When you experience menstrual complaints during your period, these yoga poses on the following pages can alleviate the pain.

Child's pose

Kneel on the ground so that your big toes touch each other, with your knees wide and your shins on the ground. Sit on your heels with your buttocks and slowly bend your upper body forward. Breathe in and out deeply. This calming and restorative posture allows you to fully relax and can help with lower back pain.

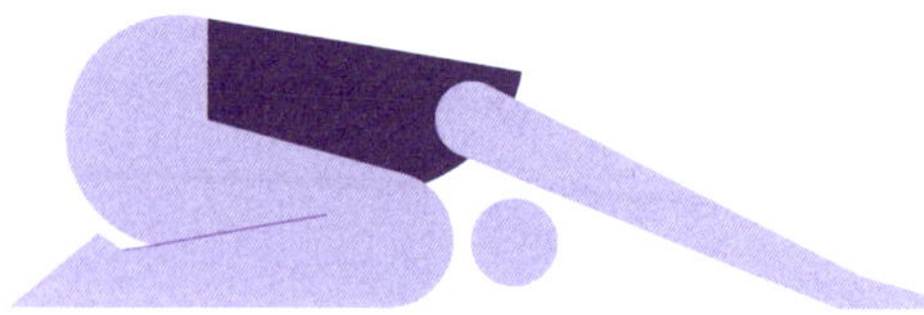

Cat-cow pose

Get on your hands and knees, with your hands directly under your shoulders and your knees under your hips. As you inhale, hollow your back, and slowly move your head back. This is the cow pose. Now exhale and arch your back slightly, while moving your head down a little. This is the cat pose. This pose is a blissful stretch and improves blood circulation, which can help reduce stomach cramps.

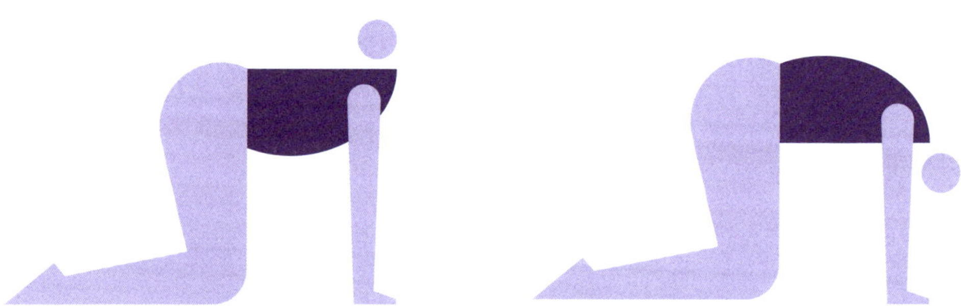

Downward dog

Get down on your hands and knees on the ground and stretch out your arms and legs, so that only your hands and feet are still in contact with the ground. Push your hips up towards the ceiling to create an inverted V shape. You can bend your knees if that feels better, and your heels don't have to touch the ground, but you do push them as far into the ground as possible. This well-known yoga pose can relieve menstrual discomfort and calm the mind when combined with the right breathing exercises.

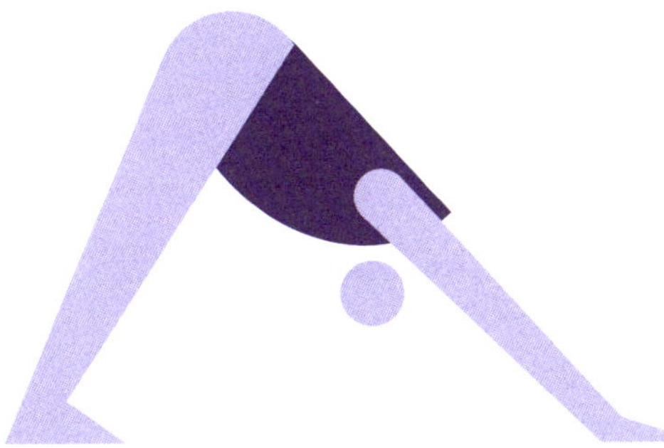

Reclined butterfly

Lie on your back, with your knees bent and your feet on the mat. Let your knees fall to both sides and place the soles of your feet together. With your arms next to your body, palms facing up, and your eyes closed, you can now take deep breaths and relax. This restorative posture opens your groins and hips. If you are experiencing abdominal cramps, a warm cherry pit cushion can be heavenly when placed on your stomach during this pose.

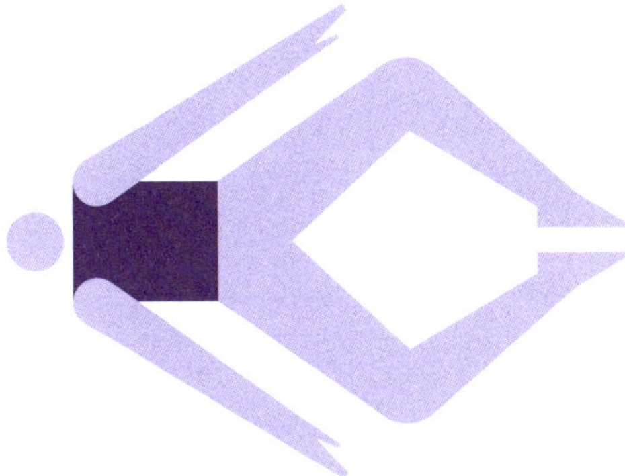

TESTIMONY

Ellen Kegels

(FOUNDER OF LNKNITS)

My two beautiful daughters were both born via cesarean section. The delivery of my first, Lucy, was induced and ended in an emergency cesarean section. The second delivery, of Lily, was a planned cesarean section, but unfortunately turned into an emergency procedure under general anesthesia immediately after the delivery. A stitch turned out to have come loose. I lost a lot of blood and was a complete wreck for months due to the constant care for the little ones and the many deficiencies in my blood.

After breastfeeding, my menstrual cycle resumed. What struck me in particular were the painful ovulations, often resulting in emergency department admissions due to heavy bleeding. What was that... This couldn't be right! I was sent away several times with only some pain medication, blood clotting agents and some 'good' advice in the form of: "This is just part of being a woman, accept it."

Cycle after cycle, I became weaker and weaker. I suffered more and more from iron deficiency and anemia. With a quarterly bag of iron via infusion, I was able to 'survive'. I lost kilos and felt terrible.

I visited several gynecologists until I finally received a diagnosis: I had a so-called "niche" or a cavity-shaped scar in the uterus. My uterus was pretty much open: fluid from ovulation and from my period seeped through my abdomen, bringing with it this huge pain with stitches and cramps.

I had never heard of a niche before. However, this occurs in half of all cesarean sections, and almost all of them in 'retroverted uteruses' like mine. This results in a constant tension on your uterus and the scar, which makes the niche or scar more likely to tear if you don't take good care of yourself or start lifting too soon after giving birth.

I quickly scheduled a first niche operation. It was during the peak of the coronavirus pandemic, so waiting times were long. I discovered Guud Woman through a colleague. The supplements could provide support against the very heavy bleeding I had, she told me. I started taking them while waiting for the surgery, and it was incredible to see how the intensity of the bleeding decreased so much.

Unfortunately, the first operation was not successful. I didn't receive sufficient information about the importance of recovery and the condition of my uterus at that time. The niche torc open again, resulting in all kinds of complaints and problems. It was dramatic. Yet I didn't let my spirits drop again: I had to and would have a healthy uterus again, with my own quality of life and my dream of another little one as my main motivators. Just FYI: a niche also greatly reduces your fertility. Although my husband is a bigger obstacle today, because he is yet to be convinced.

Luckily, after all those problems, I quickly ended up with a fantastic gynecologist, Dr. Van Kerrebroeck. She wanted to give me one last chance. She uses a completely different approach, mainly focusing on a long recovery period, so that the wound can heal properly.

The niche was excised again and beautifully sutured. The stitching itself went very well, but the uterus had become a dead mass after the many surgeries and poor self-care. It no longer had any blood circulation ... And a biopsy also determined that I had 'adenomyosis', which is an abnormal growth of endometrial tissue in the muscular layer of the uterus. Another setback. But again: where there's a will, there's a way. I delved into acupuncture and Ayurvedic nutrition to improve blood circulation. I barely moved for three months and regularly took my supplements, along with acupuncture and a warm and nutritious diet. I was also temporarily put into menopause through medication to give my uterus the rest it deserved, but I quickly stopped taking those pills because they brought me down a lot mentally. I haven't been taking hormones for almost 15 years now.

Not only did my hair grow like crazy, but my skin also radiated like never before thanks to my adjusted lifestyle. But the most important thing was that the operation was a success. The niche and adenomyosis are gone, as are my symptoms. My quality of life has improved by two hundred percent. I can exercise, take care of my family, and run my own business. Previously, it was either/or, not and/and. I continue to take the supplements every day, still go to the acupuncturist every two weeks, still eat ayurvedically, and keep mentioning my desire to have children to my husband, haha! In short, I am once again a healthy, energetic woman!

THE FOUR SEASONS
OF YOUR CYCLE

SPRING

SPRING

Spring fever caused by the first rays of sunshine, waking up while it's already light, birds singing, temperatures rising and summer getting closer, it all makes me have more energy and feel happier. The increase in estrogen also makes me feel more comfortable in my own skin, and feel like starting new projects and taking on the world again. Personally, I find that I want to spend more time with my friends, and have more energy to exercise more intensively.

Phase: the follicular phase
Duration: 7 to 10 days

Spring represents new beginnings, and that is exactly what is happening in your body. This is the period after your menstruation in which an egg matures.

The follicle-stimulating hormone (FSH) causes about 20 to 25 new eggs to grow across both ovaries. Do you remember when I mentioned earlier in this book (see p. 24) that the egg cells are stored in a fluid-filled sac or follicle? Every month, a group of follicles join the battle and they all want to take their chance to mature into fully-fledged eggs. Only one of them will come out as the winner. The dominant follicle is already selected on the fifth day of your cycle, a few days after your menstruation. The growth of the group of follicles, of which one dominates, is called the follicular phase. The follicular fluid contains a lot of estrogen, which causes your estrogen levels to peak just before ovulation. This way your body can prepare for ovulation.

HORMONAL FLUCTUATIONS DURING SPRING

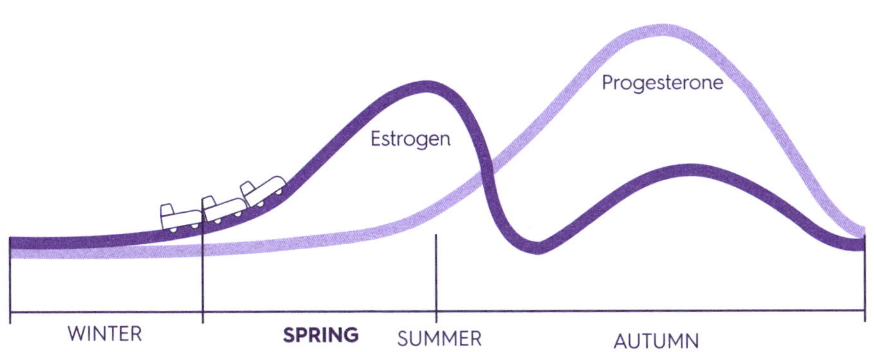

Why is this phase called spring? The follicular phase, like spring, symbolizes a new beginning. Everything is growing and blooming, including you! You probably notice that this phase after your menstruation often goes smoothly and that you are full of energy.

There is a lot happening in your body in spring, because your egg cell is maturing. You probably feel good. Your estrogen levels rise, making you feel energetic and breeze through your to-do list.

Focus on, for example:

- Everything you were putting off.
- The more challenging projects for work or school.
- Exercise! If you want, you can try to break new records.
- Enjoying yourself with friends and family.

YOUR WORK/LIFE DURING SPRING: A PHASE FULL OF ENERGY AND CREATIVITY

Your hormones are at a low level at the beginning of this phase and your estrogen starts to rise gently. This is the perfect moment to start a new project or do creative work. Plan your work ahead, brainstorm, dream big, and use your positive and creative energy in a way that is perfect for your work!

Because you have more energy in this phase, you may be able to work for a long time without interruption. Make use of this, but don't forget to take breaks on time!

YOUR SLEEP IN SPRING

Due to the increased energy in this phase, you may feel overstimulated by new ideas, making it difficult to fall asleep at times. You may also notice that you sleep lighter and that you are not really rested in the morning. The snooze button beckons...

It can be difficult to fall asleep during this phase as well as to wake up in the morning.

YOUR DIET DURING SPRING

After winter, your metabolism slows down, which means you have less appetite than in the other phases of your cycle. Choose light meals with lots of fresh and crisp vegetables and fruit. Eat enough proteins and occasionally include fermented products in your diet for a healthy functioning of the gut flora.

At the beginning of the follicular phase, your estrogen levels are still low. You can add food rich in phytoestrogens (which you can find in edamame, flaxseed, miso, tofu and soy) to your meals during these days. They can mimic the action of estrogen in your body when there is a deficiency of it. Women who experience estrogen dominance should be careful with this. Foods rich in phytoestrogens are also often recommended to women reaching menopause, as this is when estrogen levels in your body drop drastically.

I am not in favor of strict diets, but if you still want to go on a diet, it is easier to lose weight during spring. Not only do you have more energy to exercise, but you also feel less bloated and less hungry (because your metabolism slows down) compared to the week before your menstruation. Be careful, because strict dieting can have a counterproductive effect and cause stress on your body, leading to fat accumulation.

Fasting for women? Do or don't?

Is fasting the same for women as it is for men?

In recent years, there has been an increasing number of people who fast. Fortunately, this hype is also leading to more and more studies being published. I wanted to know more about the effect of fasting in women, so I consulted **Dr. Annaïk van Branteghem.**

Women and men are simply different, and, as a woman, it is not a good idea to fast in the same way as a man. If you want to fast, choose a moderate form, such as not eating for 12 hours, including the night, provided that you consume enough calories. When fasting, be sure to also pay attention to the phase of your cycle.

Women have a greater need for energy during certain phases of their cycle. Most women feel hungrier just before they have their period.

That is normal, because your body needs more calories during this period of your cycle due to hormonal fluctuations. When you fast rigorously, it can be disastrous for your (menstrual) health.

If you fast too excessively (16 hours or more), this can have an impact on your hormone production. You will produce less estrogen. This hormone is important in the first half of your cycle, when your follicles start to form. If you do not produce enough estrogen, you may not menstruate. In the long term, this can lead to fertility problems. As a woman, it is important to eat enough and take in enough calories. If you eat too little or not nutritious enough, this can have consequences for your menstrual health.

If you notice that you are experiencing an irregular cycle because you are fasting, it is better to stop. It is important to learn to listen to your body and discover what you are feeling exactly in the first and second half of your cycle.

It is not recommended for women to fast.

- when you don't have a cycle;
- when you have a desire to have a child, are pregnant or breastfeeding;
- when you have had an eating disorder in the past.

Fasting can have a positive impact on fertility with certain medical conditions, such as PCOS with obesity. Insulin resistance plays an important role here, and in this specific case, fasting can indeed provide added value. Of course, maintaining a balanced intake of nutrients (carbohydrates, proteins and fats) and a healthy number of calories remains important for a normal cycle. When you want to fast due to a specific medical condition, consult your doctor as every situation and every person is different. There is no one size fits all.

YOUR SEX DRIVE DURING SPRING

Spring is a time of renewal and extra energy, of excitement and pleasure. You are open to new experiences, so it's the ideal moment to rediscover yourself and your body. Maybe you're more in the mood for a long foreplay, or you want to try something new. Look at yourself with curiosity and openness.

You don't always have to experience sexuality with someone else, it starts with yourself. You can schedule a moment every day to connect with yourself. That shouldn't take more than five to ten minutes. You can caress or lovingly touch yourself and experience a magical moment with yourself.

Jan and I have been together for fourteen years and over the years we have grown and evolved in so many ways, but in our sex life we feel that there is still a lot of room for improvement and exploration. When you have been in a relationship for a long time, the feeling of safety and security often takes precedence over eroticism. Fortunately, we can talk about this very openly, and we still have many years to spend together and take our sex life to the next level.

Tip

Has it been a while since you had sex with your partner? Then spring is the perfect phase to grow closer to each other again. Plan a date night in and experiment with your partner. You are most open to new experiences in this phase.

YOUR SKIN DURING SPRING

Skincare advice from Marion Naudts (Marion Maakt), skincare expert: During your follicular phase, your energy level starts to rise again and your skin becomes stronger. Your skin can handle more. A perfect moment to exfoliate and remove dead skin cells. You can use, for example, a serum with fruit acids for this. Be careful not to use too aggressive serums, as they can irritate your skin barrier. A balanced skin barrier is important for a healthy skin. If you disturb this barrier too much with aggressive cosmetics, you create a breeding ground for all kinds of skin problems. So choose an exfoliating serum that is focused on both repair and balance.

EXERCISE DURING SPRING

During the first half of your cycle (from menstruation to ovulation), estrogen increases, giving you more energy, making it easier to build muscles, and allowing your body to recover faster. This ensures that you can exercise and exercise a lot every day without any problems. Spring is therefore the ideal period to spend more time outdoors, develop new skills, or experiment with new physical activities, also because you are more open to new experiences.

→ During this phase, speed and strength are the main focus. Choose strength training, intense cardio exercises, possibly HIIT sessions, dancing, cycling or swimming. If you go running, do hills and sprints.

Thanks to the scientifically supported app Wild.AI, I have learned a lot about how strength training can support your female health and the importance of keeping your muscles and bones strong as you age. As you get older, you lose muscle mass but gain fat. Personally, I do not yet have the discipline to do strength training on a weekly basis, but it is high time. Muscle mass decreases in women by approximately 3 to 8 percent per decade after the age of 30, and this rate accelerates even more after the age of 60. Now that I'm 35, it's high time to get to work. Are you joining?

Expert and personal trainer Axelle Wilssens says: did you know that strength training is good for your hormones?
Strength training has a stimulating effect on estrogen and testosterone. It promotes more muscle growth and stronger bones, which is important as you get older, because muscle mass and strength decrease. The older you get, the more important it is to do strength training. This is because women no longer produce estrogen in their ovaries after menopause. The body can only obtain estrogen through aromatase. Aromatase ensures that the body produces estradiol from testosterone. By strength training, you build muscle mass. The more muscle mass you have, the more testosterone you have, which in turn can be converted to estrogen in the body. If you suffer from PMS, strength training can help reduce your symptoms. Exercise also helps to keep your estrogen levels balanced. This is important because a low estrogen level can increase the risk of osteoporosis and cardiovascular diseases.

In your follicular phase, your estrogen rises, but so does your testosterone. This results in more strength and motivation to train, and also better recovery. During your ovulation, you are and also feel the strongest, but you are also more susceptible to injuries due to the fluctuations of estrogen that occur after your ovulation. It is therefore always important to train with the correct posture during the second half of your cycle.

Make sure you follow a good exercise routine.

- Make sure you have a schedule based on your goals so you don't do too little, but also not too much.
- Focus mainly on strength training and muscle building. In addition, you can also add some LISS (low intensity steady state cardio) for cardiovascular health.
- Start at the beginning. During training, you break down your body, and when you rest, you build muscles, cool huh? Taking sufficient rest is therefore very important, because only when you rest can your body recover and build muscle mass. Two to three times a week strength training in the beginning is definitely sufficient.
- Eat enough carbohydrates before your training. During your workout, your muscles use glucose (carbohydrates) as fuel. You should eat a meal with carbohydrates and proteins about two hours before exercising. Choose slow carbohydrates such as whole grain bread or oatmeal two hours before you start exercising, or choose fast carbohydrates such as a banana about thirty minutes before you start exercising.
- Do you exercise more than twice a week? Then your muscles need extra proteins to recover after an intensive workout. If you eat too little protein, you will find that you are less able to perform and recover. Proteins are not only important when you do (strength) training, but they are also crucial for our hormone balance. Fats and carbohydrates are sources of energy, while proteins are the building blocks of our body.

If you have no experience with strength training, I recommend that you seek guidance from a personal trainer. Never start with heavy weights if you haven't yet mastered the necessary technique. You can always practice the exercises without weights first, and once you can do them correctly, you can add weights and gradually continue building up.

TESTIMONY

Hilde De Baerdemaeker (ACTRESS)

From the age of sixteen, I started taking the pill. I was very ignorant and unprepared for the major changes in my hormonal balance at that time. It was self-evident. My primary care physician prescribed it without any problems because I had pimples and already had a boyfriend.

I took the pill until I was 32(!). It was sixteen years of intense emotional roller coasters on a relational and mental level. I suffered from severe depression and often had difficult PMS periods.

I stopped taking the pill on our pre-honeymoon, a baby was very welcome. Three months later, I was pregnant with our twins. After giving birth to the twins, I had a hormonal coil for almost a decade, which meant I had no periods for ten years.

Now, for about three years, I have been menstruating completely naturally and very regularly, without hormonal contraception. My husband underwent a minor procedure.

Because I wanted it.

Because I felt like my hormones were playing ping pong in my body and head. Because I felt like I didn't really know the real me because of that hormone roller coaster every month. That was it. Even though I had no periods during the years with the hormone IUD, I could still follow the fluctuations in mood and depressive irritable days with the calendar.

Honestly, often it was my husband who cautiously probed: "Sweetheart, where are you in your cycle?" during a monthly emotional mood. I only became angrier or sadder from it, but a few days later I had to admit it. My sensitive heavier breasts and my two extra kilograms gave away my menstrual phase.

I have still been experiencing fluctuations in the past three years, sometimes very intense ones. My system is quite hormonally regulated and I am very sensitive.

But since about a year ago, things have significantly improved. I read more about the menstrual cycle and now better understand my seasons. I take better care of myself, eat much healthier, and check more often how I'm really doing, physically and mentally. I am finally getting to know my body at the age of 44, with the help of simple notes in my agenda and a book on my nightstand. It is a mood tracker, in which I note my highs and lows alongside a monthly calendar. Very interesting to predict when the dip will come. We make it a soft PMS period by announcing in advance how I feel. Finally, we can do that. Because we have come a long way. The days when monthly heated arguments used to get the better of us are a thing of the past.

Healthy eating, meditation, indulging in the autumnal phase and a little extra hibernation during the menstrual phase, together with Guud's supplements, are a very big help for me. Those supplements really do what they promise. I notice it in everything: more peace, a clear head, a clearer skin, and a general feeling of empowerment.

When I think back to that young woman of sixteen at the doctor's, I feel a bit sad. If I could have whispered something to her back then, it would be this:

Sweetheart,

The pill may not be the right solution, it also has many disadvantages.
Try eating healthier, those pimples will improve a lot.
And you shouldn't do it for that boy.
You can be more creative than that.
Free, safe, and discover your own true self.
Take the time to truly get to know yourself, with that crazy wonderful cycle of yours. Learn to surf the waves of your emotions.
And don't think that you have to. Do whatever you want. You're doing great, I'm sure.

All love!

Yourself (from 2022)

THE FOUR SEASONS
OF YOUR CYCLE

SUMMER

SUMMER

Summer is the phase of communication and the ideal moment to discover your menstrual powers. Menstruating is always perceived as something dirty and unpleasant, but since I started living according to the seasons of my cycle, I have discovered that as a woman, you have superpowers. For example, I feel very confident during my ovulation. I can express myself better and it is easier to communicate what I really want. I also feel more attractive and enjoy spending time on my appearance. Because it makes me feel better about myself, this is the moment for me to go shopping or experiment with makeup.

Phase: ovulation
Duration: 3 to 4 days

Your egg is ready for the big adventure: ovulation or the release of the egg. The egg leaves the ovary and if there is sperm in the fallopian tubes, the egg can be fertilized there. Just before ovulation, the estrogen level in your body rises. Thanks to estrogen, your body can prepare for ovulation. Your uterine lining is building up and your cervical mucus is increasing. Did you know that you can tell if you are fertile by looking at your cervical mucus? You can read more about it on page 30.

Why is this phase called summer?
Ovulation or egg release is your fertile period. During this period, you often feel more attractive and confident, just like how you often feel fantastic with a lovely sun-kissed skin and a beautiful summer look. Everything is on fire. You probably notice that your libido is increasing, and that is no coincidence. Your body knows exactly what it's doing: thanks to a higher libido, you have more sex drive, which increases your chances of conception.

If you track your menstruation with an app, you can predict when you ovulate. You can also check your cervical mucus. Some women also feel the ovulation as a small stitch on the left or right side of the abdomen. If you have a desire to have children, this is the perfect time to have sex. And the good news is that you're probably really up for it. Your libido is currently at its highest.

The days before your ovulation, the luteinizing hormone rises and you have estrogen and testosterone peaks. The result? You feel more extroverted, sociable and energetic.

A perfect moment to:

- try something new;
- go out. Party, socialize or organize a gathering;
- have sex;
- complete a project or have a difficult conversation;
- train more intensively.

THE OVULATION PHASE

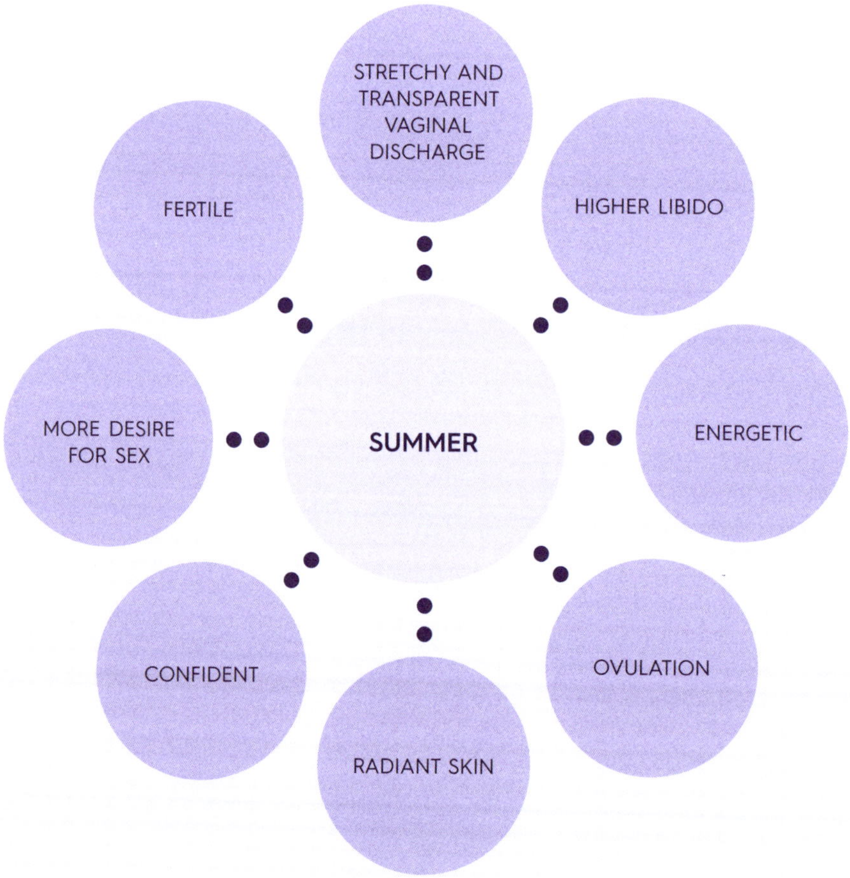

What is ovulation pain?

As if PMS were not enough, certain women can also experience symptoms or pain around ovulation. Do you feel a short stabbing pain in your lower abdomen level with your ovaries? That's called ovulation pain. The pain can sometimes be compared to menstrual pain. In addition to stabbing or cramping in your lower abdomen and lower back, you may also experience nausea and headache when you ovulate. Ovulation pain often lasts only a few hours, but some women may experience it for the entire day or even more than a day.

Different causes have been put forward for the pain around ovulation. Ovulation pain does not always coincide with the day of ovulation. You may feel that in the ovary, a mature ovary bursts open and an egg is released. Another cause is that the growing follicle can cause tension or pain in your ovary. When the egg is released, the fluid from the follicle is also released into your abdomen. Your peritoneum can become slightly irritated, which can cause menstrual-like pain. You may also lose a small amount of blood. Another possible cause of the pain is the contraction of the fallopian tube. If the pain during your ovulation is unbearable, be sure to discuss this with your doctor.

YOUR WORK/LIFE DURING SUMMER: A PHASE OF COMMUNICATION

Around the time of your ovulation, you often feel fantastic. It is a good time to have important conversations, give presentations and collaborate. You feel confident, social and happy, and you radiate this. Network, make new contacts, and definitely don't hesitate to close that new deal at work or talk to your boss about that promotion you've been waiting for so long!

YOUR SLEEP DURING SUMMER

As you could already read in the other seasons, the fluctuating hormones also have an influence on your sleep. Also in summer, all sorts of things happen. During your fertile days, you are more likely to have sexual and romantic dreams. Yes, really! In this phase, you will also feel more attractive and confident. Because your estrogen and testosterone levels are high during this phase of your cycle, your libido will cause you to have more erotic dreams. So don't feel guilty if you wake up next to your partner in the morning, but have experienced an intense orgasm with someone else in your dream. Blame it on the hormones.

A few days per month, my dreams are much more intense and vivid. As I learned to chart my cycle, I noticed that these emotional and erotic dreams often occurred around my ovulation or the days just before my menstruation. You know those dreams where you hope you didn't talk out loud in your sleep? I find it fascinating to see how my dreams vary throughout the month and how the same patterns keep recurring. When I used to dream of cheating, I always felt a bit guilty and embarrassed when I woke up next to my husband. But now I no longer feel guilty; I just blame it on the fluctuating hormones.

YOUR DIET DURING SUMMER

Summer is the most fertile phase of your cycle, during which your body prepares itself to be fertilized. The estrogen reaches its peak just before ovulation. Remember to keep your liver and intestines healthy, so that excess estrogen can leave your body properly and not remain in your bloodstream.

At the end of your summer, your body temperature rises due to progesterone. Then choose vegetables and fruits that have a cooling effect on your body. Choose foods that contain vitamin B and/or zinc. Especially zinc is important for supporting your fertility. Green leafy vegetables - such as spinach, bok choy, broccoli and Brussels sprouts - whole grains, quinoa, eggs, seeds, nuts, tomatoes, figs, strawberries, raspberries and fish are all great options to add to your meals during this phase of your cycle.

Nutrition and the quality of your eggs

Your eating habits can have an impact on your fertility and play a role in maintaining the quality of your eggs. Research shows that women can achieve improved egg quality by focusing on omega-3 fatty acids.

It is therefore important to eat enough healthy fats. Those are fats with a high percentage of unsaturated fat and a low content of saturated fat. They contain sufficient omega-3 fatty acids and little omega-6 (which you already get enough of with a normal diet).

In addition, omega-3, just like magnesium, is also important for your progesterone levels. Progesterone is one of the most important hormones for a healthy pregnancy. The production of progesterone after fertilization is extremely important. It prevents your body from rejecting the embryo, and it ensures that the uterus remains in optimal condition and that the growth of breast glands is stimulated.

You can find healthy fats or omega-3 fatty acids in fatty fish such as salmon, herring, mackerel and sardines. Not a fan of fish? You can also find omega-3 in nuts, avocado, olive oil, coconut oil, pumpkin seed oil, hemp oil and walnut oil. Organic eggs also contain good fats. Top up your reserves with a high-quality omega-3 supplement.

Per day, about 20-40% of the calories you take in should come from fat. This amounts to 44 to 89 grams of fat per day for an average woman. A few examples of healthy fats in weight:

- One tablespoon of olive oil: 10 - 13.5 grams
- An avocado: 30 - 33 grams
- 1 handful (25 grams) of almonds: 14 grams
- A portion of salmon (120 grams): 13 - 15 grams

Can nutrition increase or decrease the chance of pregnancy?
We all know that a balanced lifestyle has a positive influence on our overall health, but is there a link between nutrition and fertility? To be honest, we don't know (yet)! Research at Harvard University has not shown that the 'fertility diet' directly increases the chances of pregnancy, but it does show that it can be supportive. It doesn't hurt to try.

So give it a go!

- You can start right away.
- It doesn't cost anything.
- There are no additional negative effects.
- It is the foundation for a healthy pregnancy and a balanced diet.

So, in my opinion, it is definitely worth a try! Remember that nutrition is not everything.

Becoming pregnant is more than just eating healthy. It has to do with your age, genetics, hormones, environment, stress, not to mention your partner's lifestyle and sperm quality. All these factors play a role in your fertility. In short, you can't have control over everything, but for many things you can. Let's start with that!

- Use saturated fats and avoid trans fats as much as possible. Saturated fats can be found in nuts, fatty fish and avocado. Fatty fish species include herring, mackerel, eel, sprat and salmon.

- Choose plant-based proteins such as beans, hemp seeds, nuts, tempeh, tofu and vegetables.

- Say yes to complex carbohydrates! They have a bad reputation in some diets, but if you want to get pregnant, you have carte blanche to eat them!

- Get your iron from vegetables such as spinach, pumpkin, tomatoes, cabbage and mushrooms.

- Take prenatal multivitamins with at least 400 milligrams of active folic acid.

- Drink enough water.

- Strive for a healthy body weight. Being overweight or underweight can disrupt your menstrual cycle, possibly causing you not to ovulate.

- Exercise enough, but don't overdo it. If you exercise too much, it can prevent you from ovulating. The chance of this happening is greater if you are underweight.

It takes two to tango: men can also play their part. The same study also showed that folic acid, zinc and omega-3 can also provide added value for the quality and motility of sperm, which also plays an important role in fertilization.

YOUR SEX DRIVE DURING SUMMER

The most sexual phase for most women is in summer, when everything blooms, flows and opens up. You become aroused more quickly and you feel "all woman". You probably can't get enough of sex, whether it's in the morning, afternoon or evening. This may be a bit exaggerated, so don't panic if you don't feel like it at all, but normally that is the case because you are most fertile during your ovulation phase. Keep this in mind if you don't want children (yet)!

An orgasm is a blissful, intense and overwhelming feeling. As a young girl, I already masturbated without really knowing what it was exactly. Because I was sometimes caught by my mother, this caused a lot of shame in my upbringing. When boys start masturbating, it is considered normal. There is still a big taboo around this subject for girls. When sexuality and relationship coach Leen came into my life, my perception of sexuality completely changed. After taking a course with her, I was able to rediscover and embrace my body and sexuality.

You can only have good sex with someone else if you can bring yourself to seventh heaven. Leen: 'In the past, I often experienced pain during penetration' Many of my clients have this problem and are afraid to stop when this happens. I notice that many women are afraid to express what they like and what they don't like. Sometimes they just don't know, because they don't know their body and never masturbate. Often they are afraid of hurting their partner or being rejected if they were to ask for slower sex or breaks. Usually, there are underlying emotional patterns associated with this, with shame and sexual blocks as cause and/or effect. You can start by rediscovering and touching your body, as if you were your own lover.

It is a real pleasure discovering or rediscovering the clitoris, as there are as many as 10,000 (finally proven by research in 2022!) nerve endings flowing through it.

However, around 15 percent of women have never experienced a clitoral orgasm. But there is good news for those women. According to Leen, every woman has orgasmic potential. There are few biological or physiological reasons not to have an orgasm. There is nothing wrong with you if you haven't had an orgasm yet.

Why is it sometimes difficult then? 'That is the result of a patriarchal system in which female pleasure is less important than male pleasure, negative first sexual experiences, taboos and judgments that are passed on during up-bringing, and slut-shaming.'

The vaginal orgasm: myth or reality?
Many women, just like myself, struggle with certain sexual desires that are based on something that may not exist, namely the vaginal orgasm. For years, I have been having discussions with my husband about vaginal orgasms. I have always experienced a clitoral orgasm. But some scientists claim that vaginal orgasms actually do not exist. I was relieved that there is nothing wrong with me and that it is normal for me not to orgasm during penetrative sex. It goes like this: various studies have discovered that the vaginal orgasm is actually a clitoral orgasm based on physiology, because the clitoris also surrounds the sides of the vagina. The nerve endings in the

THE VULVA AND THE CLITORIS

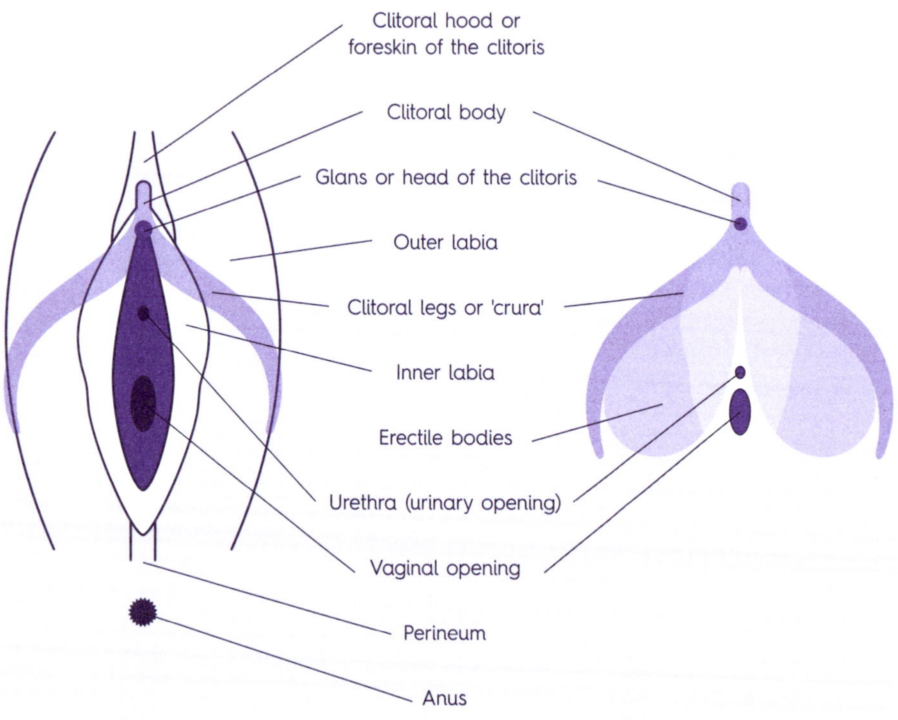

vaginal wall itself and the branches of the clitoris could potentially allow you to orgasm through vaginal stimulation, such as with a penis, dildo or fingers.

If you were to search for the magical spot for the female orgasm, search rather for the clitoris, as the G-spot is also said to be a myth. The G-spot region is described as a spongy, ribbed texture located approximately two to four centimeters deep in the vagina on the upper wall. Haven't discovered it yet? Well, you're not the only one, because there is still no evidence that this spot actually exists.

When it comes to men, only the male orgasm is talked about and that's it, while I get the impression that women are once again pressured to experience all kinds of different orgasms and that we have to climax during sex. The most important thing for me is that we can enjoy what we experience and that we learn to let go to achieve a blissful orgasm without shame or guilt. From now on, my husband and I no longer distinguish between a clitoral or vaginal orgasm, but keep it simple, just like with men, and just call it an orgasm. Like every woman, every cycle, but also every intimate moment, is unique, I don't always expect the wildest explosion when I orgasm, because by now I also know that my body and libido feel different depending on where I am in my cycle.

Did you know...

Did you know that our clitoris is actually our penis? As a fetus, we only develop our gender six weeks after fertilization. Our genitals will then start to organize themselves differently. That means that the man has the same parts as a woman. In embryology, we are all initially female. It is only when there is a testicle producing testosterone that the embryo develops further as a male, otherwise we continue to develop as a female. Yes, it's a female world! But women can also have erections because of this, although they are not as visible as with a penis. The majority of the clitoris is invisible and located beneath the skin. That is the 'crura' or the legs of the clitoris and consists of two erectile bodies. When aroused, these erectile tissues can fill with blood, causing the veins to close off, resulting in the erection of the clitoris and the labia.

YOUR SKIN DURING SUMMER

Your skin during the ovulation phase according to makeup artist and skincare expert Kim Maes from Blos shop:
During this phase of your cycle, your skin is at its best, but it is still important to take good care of it to maintain your glow.

Use a gentle facial cleanser in all stages, regardless. This removes excess sebum and impurities without drying out the skin or compromising its neutral pH. This is the foundation of beautiful skin. I like to emphasize my healthy glow even more with red lips and a highlighter in this phase.

(Kim's favorite product: Red lips: La Bouche Rouge in color: Le Doré, Highlighter: Ilia Illuminator in Cosmic Dancer)

Choose skincare products with vitamin C and hyaluronic acid, enriched with cold-pressed almond oil or argan oil for an extra boost. And if you have time, pamper your skin even more with a hydrating mask for the autumn to come.

(Kim's favorite product: Susanne Kaufmann Moisturizing Mask)

EXERCISE DURING SUMMER

Due to your reduced estrogen levels after ovulation you may feel a little weak. Do not overdo it with heavy weights, so choose lighter strength training and mainly focus on your endurance. During the summer, I usually feel at my best. I also feel more confident and sociable, which is ideal for taking a group class.

Or live it up on the dance floor, because during the ovulation phase you feel more like getting outside and being among people.

→ Choose bootcamps, CrossFit, workouts with light or moderate weights, or power yoga.

Tip

Use an app to tailor your training to your cycle.

- **FitrWoman.**
  I think this app is fantastic because it not only tracks your cycle, but also provides personal advice on exercise and nutrition. Based on your cycle, the app tells you when to push harder during a workout and when to take it easy. It also recommends foods and recipes that can help reduce menstrual-related symptoms, give you more energy, and support recovery.
- **Wild.AI.**
  Wild.AI is similar to FitrWoman. Based on your cycle and additional data, Wild.AI presents you with exactly the right workouts. In addition, you can count on nutritional advice and a supportive community. Do you think a sports app is not really for you? Well, you don't have to be a top athlete to use Wild.AI!
- **NikeSync app.**
  With the help of Stacy Sims, Nike has put together a collection of workouts that best suit the different phases of your cycle. Take day one of your menstruation as a starting point and then adjust your training to your cycle to get the most out of your workouts.

CYCLE TRACKER

Your cycle is a fantastic compass to show you the right way. Using this cycle tracker, it is easy to better understand your cycle and recognize patterns. You can keep track of various physical symptoms and feelings to better understand your cycle.

Keep track of everything for a few months and discover the power of your cycle. In this way, you will also be able to make better decisions and have a better sense of which season you are in.

TRACK YOUR CYCLE

o I have a natural cycle

o I take hormonal contraception.
Which one? ....

My cycle lasts .... days on average.

Note:
If you take hormonal contraception, you will miss certain phases that you can experience in a natural cycle. For example, you will not ovulate if you take the pill, because it is suppressed.

Examples of how you can feel during your cycle:

- Energetic
- Creative
- Tired
- Confident
- Sad
- Emotional
- Little focus
- Ugly
- Powerful

Tip: Start tracking your cycle on the first day of your period.

Month: ....

CYCLE DAY	1	2	3	4	5	6	7	... 30
Phase of my cycle (winter, spring, summer, autumn)								
Bleeding (yes or no)								
Cervical mucus (transparent, creamy, sticky, none)								
Basal body temperature								
Emotions throughout the day								
Appetite (low, high)								
How I feel during exercise								
Did I have sex? (yes or no)								
Did I drink alcohol? (yes or no)								
I feel confident / insecure								
Sleep (not good, very good)								
Feedback for myself								

CHAPTER 5

All you need to know about hormonal contraception

CHAPTER 5

All you need to know about hormonal contraception

If you use hormonal contraception such as the pill, the vaginal ring, or a hormonal IUD, then you don't have a (natural) cycle. The artificial hormones you consume daily will block your natural hormonal patterns. This suppresses your ovulation, preventing you from going through certain phases of a natural cycle. Not nothing, then.

It is often said that the hormones in contraception are comparable to the hormones your body produces, but there is certainly a difference. The hormones your body produces are natural, while the hormones from hormonal contraception are artificial.

Fortunately, you can also live cyclically, without the natural cycle. You do it like this:

- **menstrual phase**
  = the pill-free week (the days that you are not bleeding)
- **follicular phase**
  = the 7 days after the pill-free week, day 1 to day 7
- **ovulatory phase**
  = the 3 days that follow, day 8 to day 10
- **premenstrual phase**
  = the 11 days that follow, day 11 to day 21

Because this cycle is artificial, you will not experience the same benefits as with a natural cycle, but you can still feel better because of it. If you have no withdrawal bleeding when you would go on the pill or have little to no bleeding due to the hormonal coil, another option is to follow the lunar cycle to go cyclical. Then you can choose to 'menstruate' or 'ovulate' during the full or new moon.

Fact or fiction? Is the menstrual cycle linked to the moon?

The menstrual cycle and the different phases of the moon go through a cycle of about 29.5 days, which is quite remarkable. It could sometimes happen that the moon phase occasionally coincides with your cycle, but that's where it ends. Menstruation tracking app Clue compared 7.5 million natural cycles and found that the menstrual cycle does not synchronize with the moon.

The pill is one of the most well-known and widely used forms of contraception. It's ideal, because it's easy, right? But the numbers show that women are increasingly tired of taking the pill. They no longer want artificial hormones in their bodies because they want to live more naturally or they are tired of the side effects of the pill.

When using hormonal contraception such as the pill, a vaginal ring or a hormonal intrauterine device, it will affect your natural hormonal patterns. That can have an impact on your choice of partner (seriously!), sex drive, eating patterns, stress levels, appearance and mood. Sarah Hill, professor of psychology and author of the book 'This is Your Brain on Birth Control' made these findings in her research. She demonstrated that the pill has an impact on your mental health and increases the risk of depression and anxiety disorders.

What the pill does to our brain has unfortunately been insufficiently researched, but it is almost certain that the pill affects more parts of our body and mind than just the ovaries and uterus. Women who are on the pill have already indicated that they feel down and anxious, experience a low libido, or have negative thoughts. If you read the small print in the leaflet, you will see that they warn about mood swings. Unfortunately, the medical world dismisses this and we, as women, just accept it. I believe it is important for contraceptive users to receive accurate information so that they can make a more informed choice of contraception. Studies show that estradiol (a specific type of estrogen that is important during the reproductive years) influences the serotonin system and therefore plays a role in experiencing a positive, cheerful mood. When using the pill, the body produces less of this type of estrogen. In theory, this can lead to a decrease in serotonin, which can make you feel less happy. According to Hill, when there is a shortage of estradiol, the brain regions responsible for controlling anxiety are less active.

Just like Sarah Hill, I believe that women don't think enough about the effects of hormones on the brain and that they dismiss their complaints too quickly under the guise of 'it's all part of it'. What she recommends is to keep a diary when you start hormonal contraception or when you temporarily stop using it. And to ask a loved one to pay attention to any changes. Do you become quieter, more emotional, jaded? This way you can determine if the side effects of the pill are negatively affecting your life.

Is it better to choose a copper IUD then? A copper IUD does not contain artificial hormones, which means that sometimes an ovulation can still occur. The copper coil works in two ways. Firstly, copper is toxic to sperm cells, which makes them unable or barely able to fertilize an egg. Secondly, copper makes the lining of the uterus unsuitable for the implantation of a fertilized egg. Is it a good hormone-free option? Not for everyone. Unfortunately, many women experience complaints with the copper IUD because it can cause infections and inflammation. This results in severe cramps and bleeding.

The contraceptive pill has certainly radically changed the lives of women. Women finally gained control over their fertility and were able to study and participate in the labor market in large numbers. The heavy burden of not getting pregnant after sex was also finally gone, which was a relief. Just think of the many women who had to give birth in secret in convents far away from home only to never be allowed to take their newborn child in their arms in most cases and have to give it up for adoption or leave it in an orphanage. It is a dark page in our history, when women were labeled as the sole culprits in an unwanted pregnancy and their lives were forever destroyed as the only party involved. And it's not even that long ago, when you consider that the pill was only introduced in 1960.

Hormonal contraceptives do have some advantages according to gynecologist Joke Bulthé: you can plan your menstruation, you are sexually available at all times, and you can have sex whenever you want without worrying. They are very reliable in preventing pregnancy and make bleeding much less heavy, which is important for women with iron deficiency due to heavy menstruation.

But the pill, as you read earlier, has various side effects. Contraception's artificial hormones prevent an egg from maturing and being released, thus preventing you from ovulating; the cervical mucus becomes thicker and tougher, making it difficult for sperm to reach an egg; the endometrium is not built up as well, preventing any fertilized egg from settling; and you do not get your period. The blood that you lose during the pill-free week is called withdrawal bleeding. That's right, the blood during the pill-free week is not the same as menstrual blood in a natural cycle. The inventors of the pill developed it in such a way that there is a week of no pills. Therefore, the woman bleeds for a week, making it resemble a real cycle. A withdrawal bleeding is caused by a decrease in hormones in the body, because you don't take any artificial hormones during the pill-free week. You could say that it is a simulated menstruation that takes place during the pill-free week. Such bleeding is usually less heavy than menstrual bleeding, because less uterine lining is produced and therefore less needs to be broken down.

An overview of hormonal contraceptives. In short, there are treatments with one or two active hormones.

- **The pill and the vaginal ring contain two types of artificial hormones: ethinylestradiol and progestogen.** There is also the patch, which also contains estrogen and progestin. Ethinylestradiol has the same effect as the estrogen hormone estradiol and ensures a predictable menstruation. Progestagen is an artificial form of progesterone. It inhibits the release of LH and FSH and prevents the release of an egg. And if there is no ovulation, fertilization does not occur. If ovulation does not occur, your body doesn't have to 'clean up' an egg, which is why you're not really menstruating when you're on the pill or using the vaginal ring. The monthly bleeding during the pill-free week is also artificial. During the six or seven days that you stop taking the pill or using the vaginal ring, there is no intake of artificial hormones. The small amount of uterine lining that has been built up is broken down. This is called withdrawal bleeding.

- **The hormonal IUD and the mini pill contain one type of hormone: progestogen.** The Implanon implant also contains progestogen and has the same effect as the mini pill. The rod is subcutaneous and works for three years. A hormonal coil releases the hormone levonorgestrel (progestogen). This artificial hormone is also found in the morning-after pill. This hormone mainly acts on the uterine lining and causes the mucus in the cervix to become thicker. Sperm cells therefore have a harder time getting through the cervical mucus. In addition, ovulation is sometimes suppressed and the uterine lining becomes unsuitable for the implantation of a potentially fertilized egg. A small portion of the hormones from this contraception end up in your body. However, women can still suffer from the hormones that are released. Complaints include acne, mood swings, bloating and loss of libido.

DOES THE PILL HELP AGAINST COMPLAINTS?

You may have been prescribed hormonal contraception to reduce your symptoms, but unfortunately this is not a long-term solution. Because if you stop, you may experience the same complaints again. Every person is different, so the side effects of hormonal contraception can vary.

Migraine, mood swings, depression, decreased libido, gastrointestinal complaints, breakthrough bleeding, breast tenderness, unsettled skin, nausea, weight gain and a deficiency of vitamins and minerals are the most common side effects of hormonal contraception. The pill affects your gut flora, causing your organs to absorb minerals and vitamins less effectively.

I don't want to worry you or encourage you to stop using hormonal contraception, but I have used hormonal contraception for years myself and I feel a big difference between living with and without artificial hormones. But although the pill has ensured that as a teenager I no longer suffered from acne and heavy bleeding, I prefer the Morgane without artificial hormones.

Therefore, I want to provide you with insight so that you have more information to make an informed decision about what is best for you. There is still a lot of work to be done to fully understand the impact of hormonal contraception on women's health. There are fortunately other solutions than the pill to suppress your symptoms, and now you know that too!

STOP USING HORMONAL CONTRACEPTION.

What are the benefits of stopping hormonal contraception? Your feelings are no longer diminished, your natural hormonal balance is restored, you have more energy, your libido shoots up, and you feel like yourself again. But be careful, stopping the pill can also cause a lot of side effects. This is because your body is temporarily out of balance. When you stop taking hormones, your body needs to adjust to this. Your hormone balance needs to get back on track.

In one percent of pill users, it can take more than six months for the cycle to return. This percentage may not seem like much, but bear in mind that two out of five (39%) women take the pill during their reproductive years. In most cases, after about three to six months, your body gets used to the unpilling process again. At the beginning, your cycle may be irregular. Your body goes through significant hormonal changes. You can suddenly develop severe acne.

This is because the hormones in the pill suppress the production of sebum, so after stopping the pill your body compensates by making extra sebum, resulting in clogged pores and hormonal acne. If you have a lot of complaints, it may be that you are suffering from post birth control syndrome. That can occur after you stop using hormonal contraception. Symptoms include acne, amenorrhea (no menstruation), hair loss, migraines and more. Entrepreneur Nouchka De Maeyer suffered from this. Nouchka took the pill for sixteen years and in May 2022 she decided to stop taking it. Not only because she has a desire to have children in the medium term, but also because she was curious to see how her body would react without artificial hormones. She had heard rave stories from women who felt amazing after stopping the pill. They felt more connected to themselves, more energetic, happier and more feminine!

That was unfortunately not the case for Nouchka. The first two months were very tough and intense, both physically and mentally. She not only experienced pain in her lower back, abdomen and head, but also suffered greatly from depression, dark feelings and panic attacks. It even limited her ability to work. Finally at the end of her third cycle she started to feel better and decided to return to work.

But then she realized that things were actually not going that well, and she reached her lowest point. Since then, everything has accelerated: she discovered that she had post-birth control syndrome and made adjustments to her diet, lifestyle and business with the help of a nutritionist, coach and Guud Woman supplements. Since then, things have been going better.

Fortunately, she quickly got her period again after stopping the pill. Some women have to wait for months sometimes. You can see that everybody is different. Nouchka realized that by making adjustments to her lifestyle, she could indeed feel a positive difference. She has also learned that she feels different in every phase of her cycle and her emotions are no longer flattened like with the pill. By sharing her story, she wants to help other women and show them that they are not alone.

WHAT IS THE HORMONE-FREE ALTERNATIVE FOR CONTRACEPTION?

I have been using Sensiplan for a number of years now, a natural alternative to hormonal contraception. By interpreting the signals of the body during the cycle (see p. 29), the fertile and infertile days can be determined with great accuracy. The benefits of that are that you don't ingest artificial hormones, so you won't experience any of the side effects that come with it. Plus, it ensures that I also have more knowledge and control over my own body and health.

Sensiplan has been the subject of scientific research for over 35 years and is one of the most reliable sympto-thermal methods, provided that you:

- interpret the cycles correctly,
- apply the rules of the method strictly,
- you (and your partner) are motivated, and
- have high-quality guidance.

Studies at the universities of Düsseldorf and Heidelberg found that out of the 7,866 cycles examined, only three unwanted pregnancies occurred. This corresponds to a Pearl index of 0.4*. If the method is applied correctly, it has a reliability of 99.6% (method certainty), which is at least as reliable as the pill. More so, the reliability at modal use (user security) of Sensiplan is 98.2% and is said to be even better than some pill reliability studies indicate.

RELIABILITY PERCENTAGE OF DIFFERENT CONTRACEPTIVE METHODS.

HORMONAL

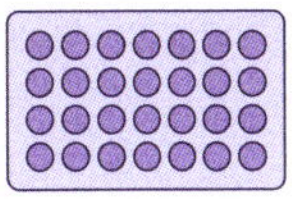

93%-99% (when used correctly)

THE PILL

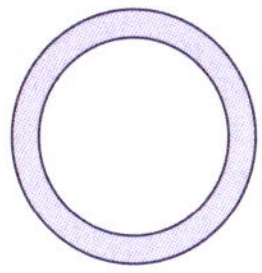

93%

VAGINAL RING

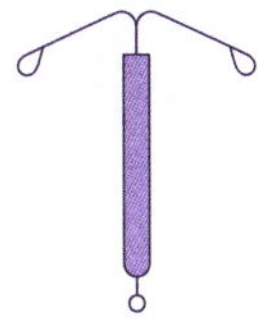

99%

HORMONAL COIL

NON-HORMONAL

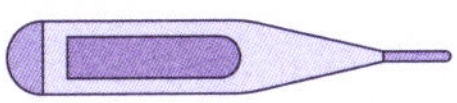

98.2%

SENSIPLAN METHOD

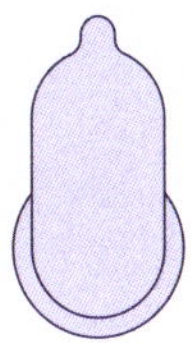

87%-98% (when used correctly)

MALE CONDOM

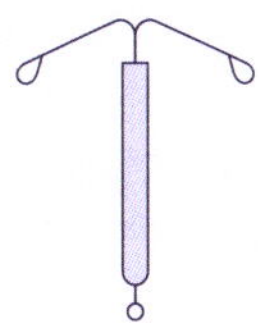

99%

COPPER COIL

TESTIMONY

Trix Eden Breuls

(PHOTOGRAPHER)

Rediscovering Myself After the Pill

Stopping the pill was a big decision, but it's one of the best choices I've ever made for myself. Since then, I feel like I'm truly me again—happier, more confident, and more in tune with my body. The change has been such a relief; I feel like I've shed both the physical and emotional weight I carried while on the pill.

One of the most exciting changes has been in my relationship. My libido surged back to life, and it's made such a difference in how connected and alive I feel with my partner. Beyond my personal life, I've noticed a positive shift in my career, too. With my confidence and energy renewed, I feel unstoppable. It's like I've reconnected with the vibrant, happy girl I was as a teenager.

While I did experience some breakouts after quitting the pill, they didn't last long. And honestly, I didn't mind—the positive changes in my mood and libido were so transformative that the skin issues felt like the smallest price to pay. I felt such a renewed sense of joy, confidence, and connection to my body that those temporary breakouts were barely a concern.

Today, I genuinely feel like I'm on cloud nine. My mood is stable, my energy is up, and I feel so much more comfortable in my own skin. I've even lost a bit of bloating and weight, which is just an added bonus. For anyone considering making this change, my advice is simple: give yourself the chance to feel amazing again.

“

I see myself blossoming again into that truly happy, confident, sexual girl - the girl I was when I was 16!

TRIX EDEN BREULS

”

INTERMEZZO

An ode to your body

For years, I struggled with self-doubt—questioning my mental health and feeling at odds with my body. This took a heavy toll on my confidence, my relationships, and sometimes even my outlook on life. I never realized that so many of these struggles were tied to my hormones and the natural rhythms of my cycle. It wasn't until I began to truly understand my cycle that I saw the connection between my symptoms and the phase I was in. Over time, I've learned to appreciate and love my body, embracing each phase as part of what makes me whole. Now, with a heart full of gratitude, I felt it was time to share this love in a letter to my body.

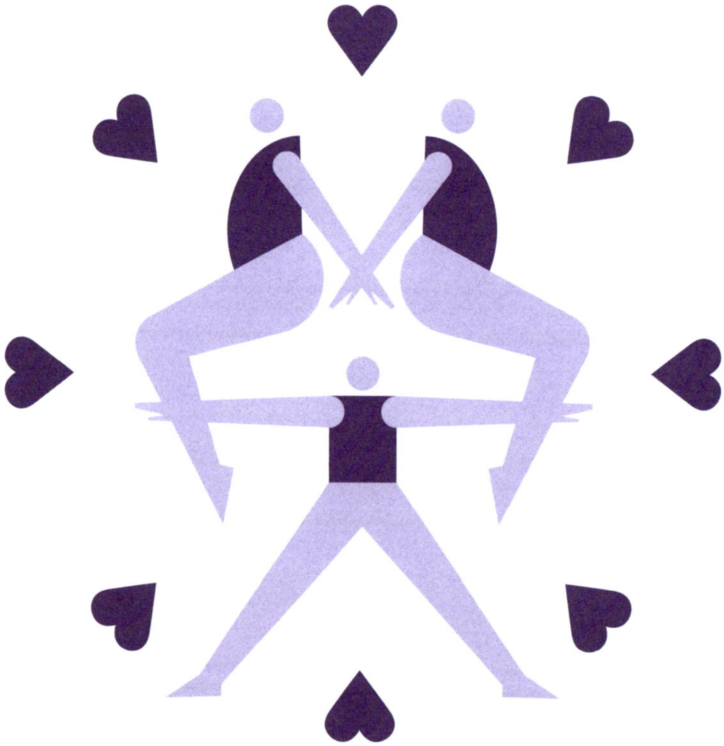

Now it's up to you. Take pen and paper, and write a letter to your body. You will see that it is liberating and also very nice to reread regularly afterwards.

Dear body,

We've been doing it together for thirty-five years. You knew me as a young girl and now also as an adult woman. So much has happened.

You were there when I traded my innocent child body for a soft woman's body with all its tenderness and curves.

You were there when my heart was first broken. You gave me tears to cry and tenderness to heal. Sometimes you said no, but I still did it. Another sip of wine. A packed schedule or lack of sleep. And yet you forgave me time and again. You knew that I still had to learn.

There was a time when I was disappointed in us. When they said I had fertility problems. When they said that you couldn't do what I thought you should do. But deep down inside, I felt that something was not right.

Because, dear body, I know you, don't I? I still know that you are there for me, that you are perfect in everything you do. And it turned out to be true. I started seeing you differently. I stood still and listened to what you said to me. You said that I had to feed you and take care of you. And little by little, I got to know you for real.

You gave me the most beautiful gift I could ever receive. I had never dared to hope for it. You let me carry our little fruit. You let my little one grow in your perfect soft warmth. We did it together. We fed it together. We are in love, together.

And, yes. Now there are sometimes folds and bulges. And veins and stripes here and there. But I have never loved you as much as I do now, my dear body.

You are my refuge, my soul and salvation.

You are gentle, warm and tender. You move, you feel, you make feel, you do. You are.

You are me. I am you. You are my everything.

Together we are perfect.

May I spend the rest of my life with you?

CHAPTER 6

When something feels wrong

CHAPTER 6

When something feels wrong

Far too many women continue to suffer from excessive pain and other complaints related to their menstrual cycle. That really needs to change. I would like to tell you that there is a good solution for each of those conditions, but unfortunately we still often remain in the dark, especially when it comes to women's health. Medical science was long based exclusively on men. Only from the beginning of the 1990s were women included in medical scientific research. They were excluded from this because of hormonal fluctuations and the possibility of becoming pregnant. Strange, isn't it? That means we have a lot of catching up to do. The bodies of women and men not only look different, they also function differently. How does it affect our health when we know that many drugs we use have only been tested on men. There are studies that show that women absorb medication differently than men. Time for change.

Fortunately, in recent years, there have been more and more initiatives to put women's health on the map. The Isala project of the University of Antwerp started a few years ago with research on the vaginal microbiome, and has produced some very interesting results. But hormonal disorders such as PCOS and endometriosis are also receiving more attention. France has even announced a national action plan to invest massively in scientific research on endometriosis. Also in Belgium, there was a hearing in the Belgian Chamber in November 2022 to raise awareness about endometriosis and discuss the gaps in knowledge about endometriosis with, among others, Prof. Dr. Tomassetti and osteopath Colette Peeters. In Spain, women are granted the right to take menstrual leave if they experience severe symptoms. However, this can be very stigmatizing for women. Personally, I don't think offering menstrual leave is a long-term solution. I am more in favor of looking at how we can prevent and reduce menstrual complaints by sharing knowledge and working together on an ecosystem where women can go for comprehensive care and guidance. That means a place where everything is bundled and women no longer have to go to separate caregivers or doctors to always explain the same problem. It would be a place where a multidisciplinary team monitors the situation and provides advice. I'm already curious about where we will be in ten years. I can already see that a lot is changing now and that more and more taboos are being broken. This allows us to have more information and take control of our health as women.

When I was diagnosed with PCOS in 2016, my former gynecologist doubted whether this was correct. According to him, this disorder only occurred in women with obesity. Although there is already a lot of information about it in the medical literature, not everyone is aware of this. This can prevent you from receiving the right help for your complaints. So, my call to everyone: if you have something that doesn't feel right or that doesn't seem normal (even if a particular doctor told you it's all in your head), search for the cause and don't give up on finding the right doctor or expert. Throughout generations, we have had to hear that certain complaints are part of being a woman, which means we don't always realize that many of those problems can be resolved.

VAGINAL YEAST INFECTIONS

I used to sometimes suffer from vaginal yeast infections. Often it was after I had had sex. So I blamed my partner and started doubting whether we were compatible and whether our pH levels were suitable for each other (blaming someone else is always easier, of course). I went to the doctor because it wasn't getting any better.

I was given Daktarin and a pill that I had to insert into my vagina. A few days later it was better, blissful! But unfortunately, these yeast infections returned regularly, even when we were not having sex. We had less sex, because if you're constantly in pain, that's not pleasant for anyone, especially not for your sex life. When I went to the pharmacist for ointment against the yeast infection, I was told that it was 'normal'. Many women experience it just before their period. I wouldn't call this 'normal'. I don't think it's 'normal' to have an uncomfortable feeling and pain and to use Daktarin for this every month.

Only later did I find out that the yeast infection and irritations were not caused by my partner, but by a hormonal imbalance. The problem mainly occurred when I was taking hormonal contraception (which I only discovered later, of course). The yeast infection only disappeared when I had my hormonal IUD removed. It took a few more months for my body to regain its balance. Since then, I have never had any more problems with monthly recurring yeast infections. There are, of course, many different factors that can cause a vaginal yeast infection, but finally I don't have to point the finger at Jan anymore, which also saves me a lot of arguments.

Apparently, three-quarters of women have experienced it at some point. A vaginal yeast infection causes itching and pain, it burns and often makes your vulva and vagina red. It is caused by the yeast Candida. What exactly happens to your vaginal microbiome has a big impact on whether or not you will get vaginal yeast infections. Because if your vaginal microbiome is out of balance, Candida gets the opportunity to multiply, causing you to experience symptoms.

Isala, a Belgian research project at the University of Antwerp, which conducts extensive research on the vaginal microbiome, has discovered that the unique composition of that microbiome and the precise ratio between the different bacteria can vary greatly. The researchers discovered that this ratio depends on the phase of your cycle, your diet, whether or not you use hormonal contraception and so much more. Also your age, the use of menstrual products, your sexual activity and whether or not you have children have a significant impact on your microbiome. They continue to analyze data, because at this moment they have been able to understand 10.4 percent of the vaginal microbiome based on the questions they have already studied.

Your vagina is generally a fantastic and harmonious place. All bacteria and yeast live in balance with one another. That is partly due to the lactic acid produced by the lactobacilli that keep your vagina pleasantly acidic. By maintaining this high acidity level, your vagina stays balanced and prevents excessive growth of yeast and bacteria. These lactobacilli and other good vaginal bacteria also produce metabolites (which are substances produced or used in metabolism), proteins, vitamins and natural products. They combat pathogens and promote health. See your vagina as a kind of factory!

Sarah Ahannach, PhD, is a doctoral researcher, microbiologist and Isala project manager at the University of Antwerp and says: 'Women are most commonly affected by yeast infections during their reproductive years. That has to do with the hormonal fluctuations of their cycle. During your cycle, your microbiome changes. Research by Isala found that women at the beginning of their cycle, in the week after menstruation, had a more diverse microbiome with more different bacteria. Women who took their vaginal samples (swabs) later in their cycle tended to have fewer different bacteria and a higher concentration of certain lactobacilli.'

Six tips to prevent yeast infections

If you suffer from a yeast infection, antifungal or fungicidal drugs (antimycotics) are usually recommended. Do not embark on this treatment without first consulting your doctor, who will help you prevent resistance and make a correct diagnosis. Prevention is better than cure. What can you do to prevent a yeast infection as much as possible?

1. **Keep your hormones in balance**
   Your hormones play a big role with respect to the Candida yeast. A good hormonal balance ensures a healthy vagina. Yeast infections usually occur around the time of menstruation. Just before menstruation, the production of the female hormone estrogen reaches its lowest point. This makes the mucous membrane layer in the vagina thinner, resulting in your vagina becoming more susceptible to yeast infections. Your pH level also plays a major role in yeast infections. During menstruation, the acidity level through menstrual blood rises from 3.5-4.5 to about 7.4! This makes your vagina more susceptible to yeast infections. You can also get a yeast infection from an excess of estrogen. This occurs around your ovulation. Bear in mind that your cervical mucus (see p. 30) changes throughout your cycle. So don't immediately assume that you have a yeast problem. During your ovulation you have more mucus or a wetter feeling in your underwear because you are in your fertile period.

2. **Adjust your diet**
   If you often suffer from a yeast infection, you can try adjusting your diet and see if you notice any positive change. For me, it definitely helped to avoid sugar, alcohol, gluten and dairy products for a few months, and to focus on a balanced diet with healthy fats, fermented foods, lots of vegetables, nuts and seeds, and low-sugar fruits. However, there is a lack of scientific evidence to support this claim.

3. **Keep your gut healthy**
   Your gut plays a crucial role in your overall health. They could also have an impact on your vaginal microbiome, also known as the gut-vagina axis. Unfortunately, we currently do not have any hard evidence for this. There are only a few research teams studying this. So just a little more patience for the connection between your gut and vagina. It can never hurt to keep your gut healthy by adding fiber-rich foods such as kefir and fermented vegetables to your diet.

4. **Do not wear synthetic underwear**
   Yeast likes warm and humid places. What I personally find very pleasant when I have this problem is to expose my vagina and vulva to the air as much as possible. I sleep without underwear at night and during the day I wear loose-fitting clothing and avoid synthetic underwear and pantyhose. I prefer to wear cotton, linen, hemp, wool or other natural materials.

5. **Try sustainable menstrual products**
   Recent research shows that the menstrual cup has a positive impact on the vaginal microbiome, unlike sanitary pads. I also prefer to use a cup or reusable menstrual underwear myself, as I am not a fan of the chemical substances in tampons and pads.

6. **Maintain your immune system**
   Some women are more prone to yeast infections when their immune system is low. There are several reasons why your resistance can have a dip. Sometimes it happens because you don't eat varied enough, or because you take certain medications like antibiotics. Also, stress can attack your immune system, so make sure you have a healthy lifestyle and avoid stress.

WHAT IS PCOS?

Polycystic ovary syndrome is a disorder of ovarian function that can lead to menstrual cycle disturbances, such as a prolonged follicular phase, irregular cycles or anovulation (when no ovulation occurs and no egg is released from the ovary during a menstrual cycle). This hormonal disorder can even lead to the absence of your menstrual periods. Often you may experience other symptoms, such as body hair and acne, which are caused by an increase in male hormones.

OVARIES IN PCOS

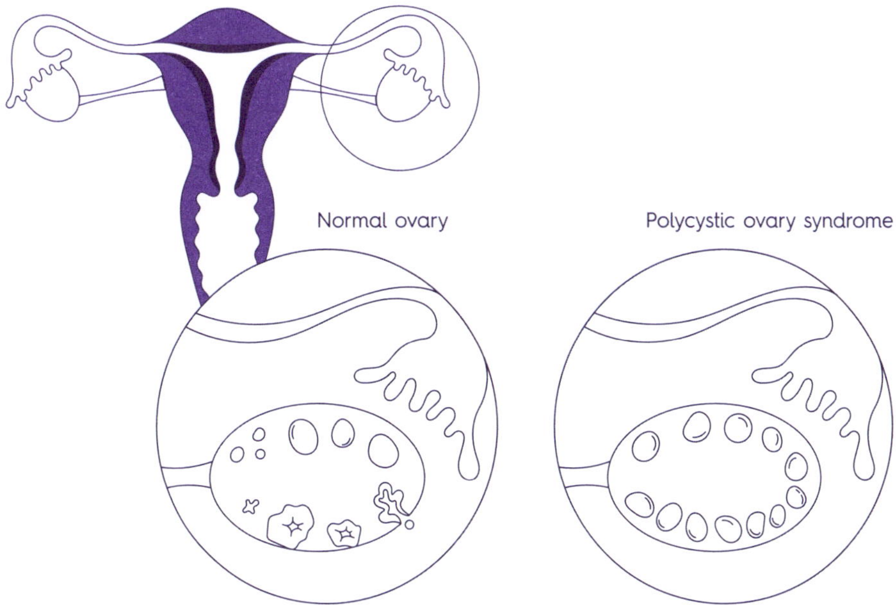

The follicular or pre-ovulatory phase lasts between seven and ten days, as the maturation of an egg varies from woman to woman. Women with a hormonal disorder such as PCOS can sometimes have a very long follicular phase (more than ten days).

After I stopped taking the pill in 2016, my periods just didn't come back. I also experienced intense mood swings and hormonal acne. I didn't feel well, so I went to the doctor. She told me that I had PCOS. About four to twenty percent of all women worldwide are said to be affected by it. In this hormonal disorder, there are many small cysts in the ovaries. Often these follicles do not grow and mature properly. This is because the level of FSH (follicle-stimulating hormone) is too low to stimulate follicle growth, and the levels of LH (luteinizing hormone) and the male hormone testosterone are usually too high. Therefore, no eggs are released and there is no ovulation. This disrupts your menstrual cycle. You have irregular periods or your menstruation is completely absent.

There are many symptoms and not every woman with PCOS has all these symptoms. The most well-known and common ones are cysts on the ovaries, weight changes, excessive hair growth (or in some cases hair loss or thinning hair), insulin resistance, oily skin and acne, and fertility problems.

PCOS and nutrition

Can PCOS be treated with nutrition? Yes, it is possible. Research shows that nutrition plays an important role in combating PCOS. A few small adjustments can already make a world of difference. Further research is needed to confirm this, but hormone coach Bénédicte De Jaeger is happy to provide a few tips. From my own experience, I can only confirm that it had a positive influence on my cycle.

We see in many women with PCOS that there is a disruption in the production of insulin. The pancreas actually produces too much insulin to keep the blood sugar level as stable as possible. In this case, we speak of insulin resistance. High insulin levels go hand in hand with excessive production of LH, which can prevent ovulation. What does this have to do with nutrition? It is important in this case to keep your blood sugar level as stable as possible. How do you do that?

- Avoid fast sugars, which are found in soft drinks, candy, cookies and many other processed products.

- Choose nutritious meals that consist of proteins, healthy fats and carbohydrates. Here are a few examples that you can easily add to your meals:

    - **healthy fats:** avocado, nuts, seeds, olive oil, fatty fish like salmon, sardines...

    - **proteins:** meat or fish, but also legumes, chia seeds and hemp seeds;

- **carbohydrates:** you can find them in vegetables and fruits, but also in grains such as quinoa, rice, potatoes and oatmeal. Furthermore, it can also help to choose gluten-free grains such as millet, barley, amaranth, buckwheat... and to reduce or avoid animal dairy products. This is to avoid additional inflammation in the body.

- If you choose a snack, opt for a piece of fruit or vegetables combined with fats or proteins, such as nut butter, seeds or hummus.

- Eat as high in fiber as possible by eating vegetables (mainly green leafy vegetables) and fruit.

- Try to exercise for at least ten minutes after the meal (walking or doing household chores)

- According to Jessie Inchauspé, who you can follow as Glucose Goddess on Instagram, it is best to consume vegetables first, then proteins, and only then carbohydrates when you have a complete meal. She is also in favor of drinking a tablespoon of apple cider vinegar with a large glass of water before meals to avoid blood sugar spikes.

Nutrition has a different impact on everyone, so individual guidance is recommended.

Exercise tips

- Do strength training: the production of muscles results in the sugars that are floating in the bloodstream being absorbed more quickly by the muscles.

- Avoid cardio: it increases cortisol production, which could further disrupt hormone balance.

- So it is best to focus on other exercise forms, such as yoga, pilates and walking.

TESTIMONY

Lynn Van Royen

(ACTRESS)

Like I think with many women, I only questioned my contraception when I started experiencing discomfort. I had a hormonal IUD and it had been working well for five years, but in the last year, it didn't agree with my body anymore. I often had stomach cramps, lower back pain, painful and sensitive breasts and nipples, and mood swings that were off the charts. Very annoying. I couldn't explain it either. Every time, I thought again: 'Oh, there's something wrong with me, what is this?' I feel incredibly down and sad. You just try carrying on, because hey, last week everything was still okay, so why not now? And even though with an IUD you don't have a real cycle, I began to discover a regularity in my feelings and discomforts.

I then posted something very open on Instagram about those hormones, and asked if they also acted up in other women. There was a massive response from women who all recognized it and had already started searching themselves. Others, like me, were just starting their search, while others generously gave advice. It felt like a warm blanket. I got to work with the advice. What kept coming back was the knowledge platform of Guud Woman and the preference for a natural cycle, which in practical terms means that you no longer use artificial hormonal contraception. In addition, I delved into specific books, podcasts and supplements to support my menstrual health. It quickly became clear that I didn't know my own body and cycle at all.

I had no idea. I had been taking the pill since I was fifteen, then I had a child, then I started taking the pill again, then I had another child, and after that I had an IUD. How would it be without? Would that still work at all? I called my gynecologist, had my IUD removed, and it felt like a huge gift to myself. Really, I celebrated the day I had my period again for the first time in six years. I was so proud that my body could still do that, that my 'little machine' still knew how to do it, that I opened a bottle of champagne with my sweetheart! I had already started taking the Guud Woman supplements before I had the coil removed. After three to four weeks, my breasts no longer hurt as much. The mood swings, on the other hand, needed a little more time, but after two months I felt much calmer. My sweetheart can confirm that. A large part of that change can be explained by the fact that I got to know myself, listened to my body and stopped contradicting my natural cycle frantically by just 'going through with it'.

When I'm in my autumn now, I am quicker to settle on the sofa. I seek out coziness, have less need to see people, and don't overdo things. I used to do that, because I thought that was expected. It's such a liberation to listen to yourself and set your own boundaries. And while I used to think: 'Oh dear, what is wrong with me, this is not at all normal', I now know that it is normal and I resign myself to it. It will pass, I embrace it. Spring and summer, on the other hand, are vibrant and bubbly! I am super social and outgoing, wonderful! Based on the season, determining your actions and behavior is enriching. We are now seven months further and every day I am happy with my decision. My sweetheart and I have also started a course at Sensiplan to know even more precisely how my cycle works and when I am fertile or not. He is also aware of everything and is part of it. In that way, he can also read me. Sometimes in the morning he says to me: 'Darling, is it possible that it's autumn?' I find that very thoughtful and sweet, and he always hits the nail on the head. That feels good, it feels like we're doing it together.

When I have my period, I like to drink infusions that have a slightly supportive effect. Herbs that can provide relief are lady's mantle, silverweed and yarrow. They work as muscle relaxants and can make your bleeding a little less less intense. And with a cherry pit pillow on your stomach on the couch, or just moving a little so that your uterus gets 'warmed up' like a muscle also helps, but that varies from person to person of course.

WHAT IS ENDOMETRIOSIS?

Endometriosis is a condition that I have no personal experience with, but unfortunately many customers of Guud Woman say they suffer from it on a daily basis. I also felt it was important to give this painful condition a place in this book, and I am very grateful that I was able to rely on the knowledge and experience of Osteopath Colette Peeters.

What is endometriosis - adenomyosis?
According to Colette, the complex condition of endometriosis and adenomyosis (endometriosis interna) is still not well-known and is difficult to recognize. However, endometriosis is said to occur in one out of nine people. The time to reach a diagnosis is very long: from seven years to more than 20 years. The lack of clear and concise information definitely plays a role.

Endometriosis is a chronic condition characterized by a hormonal imbalance. It can cause inflammations throughout the body, but especially in the peritoneum, pelvis and abdominal cavity. Even the diaphragm, the lung membranes and in some cases the sinuses can be affected. There is tissue present that somewhat resembles endometrial cells, but there appear to be more differences than similarities. The immune response and inflammation can cause adhesions, leading to organs becoming fused together. These anatomical deformities can cause a range of symptoms and often result in infertility.

Causes of endometriosis, a mystery?
Originally, it was believed that the cause was retrograde menstruation. During menstruation, most menstrual blood flows out through the vagina, but some blood can also flow from the uterus through the fallopian tubes into the abdominal cavity. This is called retrograde menstruation. Meanwhile, several hypotheses have been added to explain the cause of this disease. Unfortunately, there is no medical consensus available yet.

The cause of endometriosis, according to literature, is probably a mix of several things together: a hormonal imbalance, a genetic predisposition, an immune disorder, stem cells, peritoneal cells, harmful substances, mullerianosis (perhaps the most plausible theory, whereby the tissue would already be present in the embryo and this could develop from menarche onwards under the influence of hormones)...

It remains ultimately difficult to pinpoint a clear cause, and often various elements play a role together.

What can be the complaints of a patient with endometriosis/adenomyosis?
The difficulty in recognizing the disease is partly due to the wide range and diversity of symptoms that can have a huge impact on the quality of life. There are several functional complaints that can indicate endometriosis. The symptoms vary from person to person and are often confused with similar symptoms of other diseases, such as irritable bowel syndrome, fibromyalgia...

These symptoms include pain during intercourse (during penetration/ thrusting), gastrointestinal complaints, pain during bowel movements, fatigue, extremely painful menstruation and/or ovulation, coccyx and pelvic complaints, lower back pain, diaphragm problems, infertility, nerve pain, heavy legs, depression, reduced quality of life and more.

Pregnant women with endometriosis can also experience symptoms that are often misunderstood. Difficult postnatal recovery, for example, is not normal: this is often minimized and not recognized, resulting in a less smooth recovery for patients with endometriosis.

Adolescents and young adults can also develop endometriosis, starting from their first menstruation (menarche) and hormonal changes. Menopausal patients often experience symptoms due to old fibrotic scar tissue!

How can you diagnose endometriosis/adenomyosis?
You can recognize endometriosis based on symptoms combined with a thorough manual vaginal and anal examination, ultrasound, MRI of the pelvis and abdomen (with contrast agent), and possibly a laparoscopy with histological tissue examination. Despite improved imaging, however, not everything is visible, which means that endometriosis and adhesions cannot always be definitively ruled out based on images alone. It is crucial that an experienced and specialized gynecological surgeon performs the laparoscopic surgery. Preferably together with an abdominal surgeon/urologist/thoracic surgeon if there is a suspicion that the intestines, ureters or pleura are related to the endometriosis. Deep infiltrating endometriosis (DIE) in particular requires advanced surgery.

Everywhere pain and why?
Hormonal support, pain medication and possible surgery do not always provide complete relief of all symptoms. There are four stages of endometriosis that can be objectively diagnosed, but that does not mean that the stage of the disease is always proportional to the symptoms and pain.

Patients with a mild form of endometriosis can also experience severe pain, depending on the location of the endometriosis spots or nodules, or the strength of the adhesions that affect mobility and blood flow. Also 'central nervous system sensitization', namely the amplification of the pain signal in the brain linked to the emotional core, is important in experiencing pain.

In some patients, the pain returns over time after the surgical procedure, even though there are no new endometriosis lesions present. That is often the case with the formation of adhesions and fibrotic tissue after surgery or because a complete cleaning of certain injuries was not entirely possible. The mechanical aspect, where structures do not move supplely and elastically and thus trigger pain, can be influenced by internal and abdominal osteopathic techniques to improve range of motion.

Delaying surgery can increase the risk of anatomical deformity of the reproductive organs, with a higher likelihood of developing pain and fertility problems. Therefore, it is extremely important to include endometriosis in the differential diagnosis in adolescents as well. Differential diagnosis is a scientific method to establish a diagnosis from a list of possible conditions that a certain patient could be suffering from, given the complaints and symptoms that are known at that moment. Due to a lack of adequate knowledge among doctors, healthcare providers and patients, patients have been suffering in silence for years.

Endometriosis and fertility?
Endometriosis is often associated with fertility problems. However, not all patients with the condition will necessarily have difficulties getting pregnant naturally. The degree, severity and location of endometriosis are among the factors that play a role in fertility. In any case, each patient will require a personalized approach tailored to their specific issues.

What treatments are recommended for a patient with endometriosis?
Unfortunately, there is still no treatment to cure the disease. To date, the main focus has been on managing complaints and treating any fertility problems (if there is a desire to have children). These treatments consist of administering painkillers and/or hormonal therapy, and/or a surgery in which the endometriosis tissue, chocolate cysts and adhesions are removed. There are various medications that primarily intervene in the menstrual cycle or relieve pain. It is important to realize that there is no medication that makes endometriosis disappear.

When there is severe damage and infiltrated fibrotic lesions, it is sometimes necessary to remove part of an organ or an entire organ. This can be a piece of intestine, an ovary or the uterus. That is not done because it can cure endometriosis; it simply reduces the pain symptoms. In addition to these regular treatment methods, internal osteopathic techniques, stretching exercises, hydrotherapy and lifestyle changes can also have positive effects on the quality of life of patients, and therefore are of demonstrable value.

Colette Peeters is an osteopath (D.O., Msc.) with expertise in gynecological conditions such as endometriosis, and over the years has been able to refer and help many women just like Nina.

Since her early teenage years, Nina has been experiencing severe pain during her periods. This has only got worse as she got older. Endometriosis was a well-known phenomenon in her family, so she had already gone to the gynecologist on her own initiative at the age of thirteen. The pain was never taken seriously and she was sent home every time because the ultrasounds showed 'nothing unusual'. This continued until she coincidentally ended up visiting Colette Peeters due to another injury. After her first appointment, Colette took the pain seriously and immediately referred her for a laparoscopy, which led to the endometriosis diagnosis. Since then, she has been receiving treatment from Colette. There is no longer any severe pain. Previously, it was not possible for her to be sexually active due to the pain. Bowel movements were difficult and she constantly felt her stomach bloated. This is all in the past now! Thanks to the treatments, she can be sexually liberated again and no longer feels that having children is an impossible mission. Thanks to Colette, she was able to pick up her life without pain and fortunately received an early diagnosis. This has saved her a lot of misery and sadness.

Manual therapies such as internal osteopathic techniques (vaginal or rectal) and external osteopathic techniques applied by Colette according to WHO Benchmarks (2010) are essential both pre- and postoperatively in the examination and treatment of functional complaints and complications associated with endometriosis and adhesions. Studies show that osteopathic techniques have positive effects on the quality of life of patients with endometriosis.

Colette works closely in a multidisciplinary fashion with gynecologists, abdominal surgeons and urologists to treat each endometriosis patient according to their individual needs. A great example of how conventional and complementary medicine can work together to improve the patient's quality of life.

“Living according to my cycle allows me to feel even more at home in my body, fully connecting with who I truly am.”

Morgane Leten

CHAPTER 7

What comes after your fertile period? The (peri) menopause

CHAPTER 7

What comes after your fertile period? The (peri)menopause

I can imagine that menopause seems like a distant concern when you're in your twenties, thirties or forties, and something you don't have to worry about yet. But believe me, you are better off being well prepared so that the transition goes smoothly. The menopause is still very much a taboo subject, and I can imagine that there are few women who experience this as a pleasant time. Still, understanding your body can make this transition a lot easier.

The time before the menopause is called the perimenopause. It literally means 'around the menopause'. It is the phase in your life where your body starts preparing for menopause, and it signals the end of your reproductive years. This phase is a period of transition, and usually starts a few years before the actual menopause. For some women, this can already start around their forties. The ovaries then slowly stop producing hormones, which causes the first symptoms of menopause to appear. When you have not menstruated for a year, you are in menopause.

Typical characteristics of perimenopause:

- irregular cycles (after possibly having regular menstruation for years);
- lighter or heavier menstruation;
- weight gain;
- low libido;
- PMS symptoms;
- hot flashes or night sweats.

Unfortunately, your menopausal symptoms can be severe if you experience a lot of PMS symptoms during your reproductive phase. By getting to know your cycle during the reproductive phase and knowing how to alleviate certain symptoms through small adjustments in your lifestyle, you will certainly be grateful that you invested time in this now.

Seven tips from Bénédicte De Jaeger (Hormonal Coach)

The better you monitor your symptoms during the reproductive years, the easier and smoother the transition will be.

1. **Healthy fats and proteins are always central.** Make sure you eat the three macronutrients with every main meal, as well as with your snacks. By combining carbohydrates with proteins and fats, you ensure a more stable blood sugar level.
2. **Have foods with omega-3 on the menu often**, such as salmon, sardines, tuna, walnuts and flaxseed, or take a supplement if you find it difficult to get enough omega-3 through your diet. It is the foundation of a healthy hormone balance, because hormones are made from fats. During perimenopause, this is especially important because studies have shown that omega-3 helps reduce mood swings, depression and hot flashes.
3. **Put plenty of calcium-rich foods on the table.** For example: almonds, broccoli, green leafy vegetables, dairy, oranges, sardines and sweet potatoes. If you continuously have enough calcium, this will reduce your risk of osteoporosis (bones lose density) during the (peri)menopause. And did you know that you absorb calcium better when you have enough vitamin D in your body?

4. **Try to reduce stress or find a way to deal with it.** Chronic stress can actually cause you to enter menopause prematurely. It eventually causes the gonadal axis (hypothalamus-pituitary-adrenal axis) to close, resulting in irregular menstrual cycles which stop in the end.
5. As you get **older**, your body will need about **fifty percent more proteins** than that of a younger adult. This is because your body absorbs proteins less efficiently. Proteins are important for maintaining your muscle mass, strength and overall quality of life. Consuming enough proteins also helps to strengthen your immune system and shorten the recovery time from inflammations. If you think you're not getting enough protein, consider taking a plant-based protein powder. You can easily add it to smoothies or yogurt in the morning.
6. **Do strength training**: it compensates for progressive muscle loss and keeps the bones strong. The older you get, the harder it is to build muscle mass. You better start young to prepare for the transition.
7. Your body needs **more vitamins and minerals** as you get **older**, such as folic acid, vitamin B's, omega-3 and magnesium. If you do not get enough of these nutrients from food, take supplements.

I am not afraid of the (peri)menopause. Since I have been living according to my natural cycle, I have come to know my body well and have also learned to cope with my symptoms. Thanks to small adjustments in my lifestyle combined with the right supplements, I have been able to reduce my symptoms and some have even completely disappeared. I am convinced that as a result I will never need artificial hormones again to stabilize my hormones. Sometimes I find it crazy that we are prescribed artificial hormones for our entire lives as if this is the only solution.

If you are a teenager who has just started menstruating and you experience symptoms such as heavy bleeding, an irregular cycle or acne, you will be prescribed the pill. After years of taking hormonal contraception, you consider stopping because you may want to have children. Since I have been living according to my natural cycle, I have come to know my body well and have also learned to cope with my symptoms. After pregnancy, you quickly go back on the pill, because after all, you don't want to take the risk of an unwanted pregnancy. And when menopause approaches, you are offered hormone therapy (with various side effects such as sexual problems, weight gain, sadness and depression, but we just accept this). I compare the female existence to foie gras. We are being stuffed until we drop. This is the moment to take action and discover the power of your cycle. Take the time to walk this path. Surround yourself with your partner or friends who support you in this, or seek the help of an expert who can guide you in the right direction. You don't have to make big changes. Take small steps day by day, week by week, and month by month. Discover the options you have and make better decisions, so that you feel good every day of the month.

TESTIMONY

Kim Clijsters (FORMER PROFESSIONAL TENNIS CHAMPION)

I recently turned 41 and, like many women my age, I've started noticing shifts in my body. Some days, I feel as energized as I did in my twenties, but then there are those other days when I'm left wondering: what's going on?

At first, it was limited to small changes: brain fog, hot flashes, a bit of weight gain and feeling tired. These symptoms left me feeling off balance and questioning what was happening to me. I talked to friends about it, and that's when I first heard the terms 'menopause' and 'perimenopause'. I began researching, listening to podcasts, and connecting the dots. It was such a relief to know that this wasn't just in my head but something real that so many women experience.

Thanks to my long tennis career, I've learned to listen to my body and take good care of it. Whether it was fine-tuning my diet, monitoring my energy levels, or adjusting my routines, I developed a mindset of curiosity and self-care. Now, I've adapted those habits to support me during this new phase. For example, I prepare fresh-cooked meals tailored to my cycle, using different ingredients depending on which stage I'm in. I've also added fermented foods to my daily meals, which have helped my digestion and overall vitality. During my morning walks, I combine movement with learning through listening to podcasts. It's a moment to stay active while expanding my knowledge on various topics. I prioritize rest by going to bed early, and I make time for self-care practices like relaxing in the sauna. All of these small adjustments help me feel more balanced and in tune with my body.

Now, that same approach helps me look at this new life stage with curiosity rather than fear. I see perimenopause as just another part of getting to know myself better and embracing my body as it evolves.

To all the women out there who might feel misunderstood or struggle with unexpected shifts in energy and mood – know that you're not alone. There's still so much we don't openly discuss about this stage of life, and I hope that by sharing my story in the podcast *Beyond the Cycle*, I can help trigger more conversations. There's a quiet strength in understanding, and as I continue to learn, I'm eager to enter this new chapter with acceptance and self-compassion.

Let's remember to be gentle with ourselves. Embrace the changes, seek support, and know that you deserve to feel heard and seen.

DECODE
YOUR CYCLE

Thank you

Thank you

This book would never have existed without the help and knowledge of many others.

First of all, I want to thank you as a reader for buying and reading this book. Hopefully this book will inspire you to use your cycle to your advantage and to empower yourself, because you have the right to feel good every day of the month.

In addition to you as a reader, I would like to thank a few other people.

In particular, Yasmine, Eline and Sofie from Lannoo Publishing. Thank you for giving me the opportunity to write this book. You have helped me tremendously in developing the idea and perfecting the final version. I would also like to thank Sherita for writing this book with me in the beginning. You helped set me on the right path.

To my husband Jan, my greatest support, the best dad and my dearest partner for life. I have learned to dare to dream big thanks to you, and you ensure that my plans and ideas become reality. I am very proud that we have founded Guud Woman together, and that as a man you know so much about the cycle and support me in this. I can't imagine a better co-pilot on this roller coaster.

Thanks to my son Richard. Six years ago, I was told that it would be difficult to get pregnant, and suddenly there you were... completely unplanned. You made me realize that I had little knowledge about my body and cycle. It was only from the moment you were here that I started to delve into the cycle and how my lifestyle affects it.

Thank you to Sayrade and my sister Coralie for all the messages and support in their various forms. You have always supported everything I do since the beginning.

Thanks to Tina and Zinzi for giving the book more color and shape.

Thank you to all the wonderful women who have written a testimonial. I am convinced that by sharing your story, you can help other women and make them feel less alone.

Thank you to all the experts for sharing knowledge and shaping the book, so that we can provide the right information for women to make better decisions and take control of their health. Special thanks to Rebecca and Colette for proofreading everything.

Sources

Sources

Anticonceptiepil. (2022, 1 november). Apotheek.nl. https://www.apotheek.nl/zorg-van-de-apotheker/uw-apotheker-geeft-antwoord/anticonceptiepil#werking-anticonceptiepil

Aujla, R. (2019). The Doctor's Kitchen - Eat to Beat Illness: *A Simple Way to Cook and Live the Healthiest, Happiest Life. Thorsons.*

Baker, F. C., & Lee, K. A. (2018). Menstrual Cycle Effects on Sleep. *Sleep Medicine Clinics, 13*(3), 283–294. https://doi.org/10.1016/j.jsmc.2018.04.002

Bakker, E. B. (n.d.). *Connection Between Chronic Yeast Infections And Hormonal Imbalance.* YeastInfection.Org. https://www.yeastinfection.org/connection-between-chronic-yeast-infections-and-hormonal-imbalance/

Bauer, J. M., Biolo, G., Cederholm, T., Cesari, M., Cruz-Jentoft, A. J., Morley, J. E., Phillips, S. M., Sieber, C. C., Stehle, P., Teta, D., Visvanathan, R., Volpi, E., & Boirie, Y. (2013). Evidence-Based Recommendations for Optimal Dietary Protein Intake in Older People: A Position Paper From the PROT-AGE Study Group. *Journal of the American Medical Directors Association, 14*(8), 542–559. https://doi.org/10.1016/j.jamda.2013.05.021

Bayer. (z.d.). *Bijsluiter Mirena-spiraal.* https://db.cbg-meb.nl/bijsluiters/h16681.pdf

Bayer, J., Bandurski, P., & Sommer, T. (2013). Differential modulation of activity related to the anticipation of monetary gains and losses across the menstrual cycle. *European Journal of Neuroscience, 38*(10), 3519–3526. https://doi.org/10.1111/ejn.12347

Bradshaw, H. K., Mengelkoch, S., & Hill, S. E. (2020). Hormonal contraceptive use predicts decreased perseverance and therefore performance on some simple and challenging cognitive tasks. *Hormones and Behavior, 119*, 104652. https://doi.org/10.1016/j.yhbeh.2019.104652

Broach, J. R. (2012). Nutritional Control of Growth and Development in Yeast. *Genetics, 192*(1), 73–105. https://doi.org/10.1534/genetics.111.135731

Brody, S. (2010). The Relative Health Benefits of Different Sexual Activities. *The Journal of Sexual Medicine, 7*(4), 1336–1361. https://doi.org/10.1111/j.1743-6109.2009.01677.x

Brønnick, M. K., Økland, I., Graugaard, C., & Brønnick, K. (2020). The Effects of Hormonal Contraceptives on the Brain: A Systematic Review of Neuroimaging Studies. Frontiers in Psychology, 11. https://doi.org/10.3389/fpsyg.2020.556577

Burlison, S. (2018). *The Gut Paradox: Could Digestive Health Be the Root Cause of Most Health Problems Ranging from Hormone Issues, Autoimmune Disorders and Even Cancer?* Bookbaby.

Campbell, L. (2021, January 19th). Why Doctors Consider Your Period the Fifth Vital Sign of Health (By Veracity). Veracity Selfcare. https://veracityselfcare.com/knowledge/body/period-fifth-vital-sign?gclid=Cj0KCQjwvZCZBhCiARIsAPXbajuHdafXfKuAHc7nKpu8tWbaD6wM9ZpaFS-cAUkCBVXSmFPmf8_NMPoaAgIIEALw_wcB

Chhabra, S. (2021). Yoga Therapy for Treatment of Menstrual Disorders without Obvious Causes. *Journal of Yoga and Physiotherapy, 8*(5). https://doi.org/10.19080/jyp.2021.08.555747

De Jonge, X. A. K. J., Thompson, M. W., Chuter, V., Silk, L., & Thom, J. M. (2012). Exercise Performance over the Menstrual Cycle in Temperate and Hot, Humid Conditions. *Medicine and Science in Sports and Exercise, 44*(11), 2190–2198. https://doi.org/10.1249/MSS.0b013e3182656f13

De Weijer, T. (2021). *Eet beter voor je maag en darmen met huisarts Tamara de Weijer: met huisarts Tamara de Weijer.* Kosmos Uitgevers.

Demir, A., Uslu, M. E., & Arslan, O. E. (2016). The effect of seasonal variation on sexual behaviors in males and its correlation with hormone levels: a prospective clinical trial. *Central European Journal of Urology, 69*(3), 285–289. https://doi.org/10.5173/ceju.2016.793

Deswal, R., Narwal, V., Dang, A. S., & Pundir, C. S. (2020). The Prevalence of Polycystic Ovary Syndrome: A Brief Systematic Review. *Journal of Human Reproductive Sciences, 13*(4), 261. https://doi.org/10.4103/jhrs.jhrs_95_18

Diekhof, E. K., & Ratnayake, M. (2016). Menstrual cycle phase modulates reward sensitivity and performance monitoring in young women: Preliminary fMRI evidence. *Neuropsychologia, 84*, 70–80. https://doi.org/10.1016/j.neuropsychologia.2015.10.016

Dubey, N., Hoffman, J. A., Schuebel, K. E., Yuan, Q., Martinez, P., Nieman, L. K., Rubinow, D. R., Schmidt, P., & Goldman, D. (2017). The ESC/E(Z) complex, an effector of response to ovarian steroids, manifests an intrinsic difference in cells from women with premenstrual dysphoric disorder. *Molecular Psychiatry, 22*(8), 1172–1184. https://doi.org/10.1038/mp.2016.229

Dupont, J., Dedeyne, L., Dalle, S., Koppo, K., & Gielen, E. (2019). The role of omega-3 in the prevention and treatment of sarcopenia. *Aging Clinical and Experimental Research, 31*(6), 825–836. https://doi.org/10.1007/s40520-019-01146-1

Fathizadeh, N., Ebrahimi, E., Valiani, M., Tavakoli, N., & Yar, M. H. (2010). Evaluating the effect of magnesium and magnesium plus vitamin B6 supplement on the severity of premenstrual syndrome. *Iranian journal of nursing and midwifery research, 15*(Suppl1), 401–405. https://www.ncbi.nlm.nih.gov/pmc/articles/PMC3208934/

Fauser, B., Bogers, J., & Drogendijk, A. (1990, 18 februari). *Hormonale regulatie van follikelrijping en ovulatie.* NTvG. https://www.ntvg.nl/artikelen/hormonale-regulatie-van-follikelrijping-en-ovulatie

Fenster, L., Quale, C., Waller, K., Windham, G. C., Elkin, E. P., Benowitz, N. L., & Swan, S. H. (1999). Caffeine Consumption and Menstrual Function. *American Journal of Epidemiology, 149*(6), 550–557. https://doi.org/10.1093/oxfordjournals.aje.a009851

Freeman, E. W., Sammel, M. D., Rinaudo, P. J., & Sheng, L. (2004). Premenstrual Syndrome as a Predictor of Menopausal Symptoms. *Obstetrics & Gynecology, 103*(5, Part 1), 960–966. https://doi.org/10.1097/01.aog.0000124804.81095.7f

Hamilton, L. D., & Meston, C. M. (2014). Chronic Stress and Sexual Function in Women. *The Journal of Sexual Medicine, 10*(10), 2443–2454. https://doi.org/10.1111/jsm.12249

Hamilton, L. D., Rellini, A. H., & Meston, C. M. (2008). Cortisol, Sexual Arousal, and Affect in Response to Sexual Stimuli. *The Journal of Sexual Medicine, 5*(9), 2111–2118. https://doi.org/10.1111/j.1743-6109.2008.00922.x

Gaskins, A. J., & Chavarro, J. E. (2017). Diet and fertility: a review. *American Journal of Obstetrics and Gynecology, 218*(4), 379–389. https://doi.org/10.1016/j.ajog.2017.08.010

Groves, M. N. (2016). *Body into Balance: An Herbal Guide to Holistic Self-Care*. Storey Publishing.

Guay, A. T., & Jacobson, J. (2002). Decreased Free Testosterone and Dehydroepiandrosterone-sulfate (DHEA-S) Levels in Women with Decreased Libido. *Journal of Sex & Marital Therapy, 28*(supl), 129–142. https://doi.org/10.1080/00926230252851258

Guillermo, C. J., Manlove, H. A., Gray, P. H., Zava, D. T., & Marrs, C. (2010). Female social and sexual interest across the menstrual cycle: the roles of pain, sleep and hormones. *BMC Women's Health, 10*(1). https://doi.org/10.1186/1472-6874-10-19

Haller, D. (2018). *The Gut Microbiome in Health and Disease*. Springer.

Hantsoo, L., & Epperson, C. N. (2015). Premenstrual Dysphoric Disorder: Epidemiology and Treatment. *Current Psychiatry Reports, 17*(11). https://doi.org/10.1007/s11920-015-0628-3

Harvard Health. (August 9, 2022). Perimenopause: *Rocky road to menopause*. https://www.health.harvard.edu/womens-health/perimenopause-rocky-road-to-menopause

Hassan, I. A., Ismail, K. M. K., & O'Brien, S. (2004). PMS in the perimenopause. *Journal of the British Menopause Society, 10*(4). https://doi.org/10.1258/136218004272111

Heaney, R. P., & Layman, D. K. (2008). Amount and type of protein influences bone health. *The American Journal of Clinical Nutrition, 87*(5), 1567S-1570S. https://doi.org/10.1093/ajcn/87.5.1567s

Heineman, M. J. (2012). *Obstetrie en gynaecologie: De voortplanting van de mens* (7de editie). Springer Media B.V.

Herbenick, D., Fu, T., Arter, J., Sanders, S. A., & Dodge, B. (2017). Women's Experiences With Genital Touching, Sexual Pleasure, and Orgasm: Results From a U.S. Probability Sample of Women Ages 18 to 94. *Journal of Sex & Marital Therapy, 44*(2), 201–212. https://doi.org/10.1080/0092623x.2017.1346530

Hevigbloedverlies. (2022, 18 juli). *Aandacht voor een bloedserieus probleem - Hevigbloedverlies*. Hevigbloedverlies.nl. https://www.hevigbloedverlies.nl/bloedserieus/

Hirotsu, C., Tufik, S., & Andersen, M. L. (2015). Interactions between sleep, stress, and metabolism: From physiological to pathological conditions. *Sleep Science, 8*(3), 143–152. https://doi.org/10.1016/j.slsci.2015.09.002

Huhtaniemi, I. (2014). Andropause - lessons from the European Male Ageing Study. *Annales D Endocrinologie, 75*(2), 128–131. https://doi.org/10.1016/j.ando.2014.03.005

Hyman, M. (2023). *Young Forever: The Secrets to Living Your Longest, Healthiest Life*. Little, Brown Spark.

Isabel, J. (2020, 17 april). *Je bloedsuikerspiegel en menstruatieklachten (oestrogeendominantie)*. De Krachtige Vrouw. https://www.dekrachtigevrouw.com/post/je-bloedsuikerspiegel-en-menstruatie-klachten-oestrogeendominantie

Isala. (n.d.). *Information for medical professionals*. https://isala.be/en/information-for-medical-professionals/

Jehan, S., Auguste, E., Hussain, M. M., P., Brzezinski, A., Gupta, R., Attarian, H., Jean-Louis, G., & McFarlane, S. I. (2016). Sleep and Premenstrual Syndrome. *Journal of Sleep Medicine and Disorders, 3*(5), 1061. https://pubmed.ncbi.nlm.nih.gov/28239684/

Khalili, H. (2016). Risk of Inflammatory Bowel Disease with Oral Contraceptives and Menopausal Hormone Therapy: Current Evidence and Future Directions. *PubMed Central, 39*(3), 193–197. https://doi.org/10.1007/s40264-015-0372-y

Lande, S. (November 10, 2022). *The Clitoris Steps Into the Spotlight With New Scientific Discovery*. WebMD. https://www.webmd.com/women/news/20221110/clitoris-steps-into-the-spotlight-major-scientific-discovery

Lebeer, S., Ahannach, S., Wittouck, S., Gehrmann, T., Eilers, T., Oerlemans, E., Condori, S., Dillen, J., Spacova, I., Donck, L. V., Masquiller, C., Bron, P. A., Van Beeck, W., De Backer, C. J. S., Donders, G., & Verhoeven, V. (2022). Citizen-science map of the vaginal microbiome. *Research Square*. https://doi.org/10.21203/rs.3.rs-1350465/v1

Lee, Y., & Im, E. (2016). Stress and Premenstrual Symptoms in Reproductive-Aged Women. *Health Care for Women International, 37*(6), 646–670. https://doi.org/10.1080/07399332.2015.1049352

Lotties Period Underwear. (2020, 2 december). *Waarom je tijdens je menstruatie suiker beter kan laten liggen*. https://lottiesperiod.com/lichaam/tijdens-je-menstruatie-die-chocoladereep-beter-kan-laten-

Man, A., Ciurea, C. N., Păsăroiu, D., Savin, A. I., Toma, F., Sular, F., Santacroce, L., & Mare, A. (2017). New perspectives on the nutritional factors influencing growth rate of Candida albicans in diabetics. An in vitro study. *Memorias Do Instituto Oswaldo Cruz, 112*(9), 587–592. https://doi.org/10.1590/0074-02760170098

Mateo, A. (July 14, 2022). *Is Your Sugar Habit the Cause of Chronic Yeast Infections?* Health. https://www.health.com/condition/yeast-infection/does-sugar-cause-yeast-infections#:~:text=Sugar%20and%20the%20Body&text=%22When%20there's%20too%20much%20sugar,Shepherd.

Mawet, M. (2016, 28 januari). *De hormonen van de menstruatiecyclus* (Door Gyn & Co). Gyn&co. https://www.gynandco.be/nl/de-hormonen-van-de-menstruatiecyclus/

Menstrual Cycle May Change Women's Brains. (May 16, 2005). WebMD. https://www.webmd.com/women/news/20050516/menstrual-cycle-may-change-womens-brains

Meulenberg, R. (2018, 4 april). *Wat is DHEA?* Meulenberg Training en Coaching. https://ruudmeulenberg.nl/stress/dhea/

Milart, P., Woźniakowska, E., & Wrona, W. (2018). Selected vitamins and quality of life in menopausal women. *Przeglad Menopauzalny, 17*(4), 180–184. https://doi.org/10.5114/pm.2018.81742

Mindbodygreen, Jardim, N., & Trubow, W. (January 29, 2020). *5 Signs You Have A Healthy Menstrual Cycle*. mindbodygreen. https://www.mindbodygreen.com/0-16043/5-signs-you-have-a-healthy-menstrual-cycle.html

Mohammed, L., Jha, G., Malasevskaia, I., Goud, H. K., & Hassan, A. (2021). The Interplay Between Sugar and Yeast Infections: Do Diabetics Have a Greater Predisposition to Develop Oral and Vulvovaginal Candidiasis? *Cureus, 13*(2), e13407. https://doi.org/10.7759/cureus.13407

Moorman, I. R. (2022a, augustus 30). *Testosteron hormoon*. De Hormoonfactor. https://www.dehormoonfactor.nl/testosteron-hormoon

Moorman, I. R. (2022b, september 29). *Slaapproblemen*. De Hormoonfactor. https://www.dehormoonfactor.nl/slaapproblemen

Newson, L. (n.d.). *Premenstrual syndrome and menopause*. Balance. https://www.newsonhealth.co.uk/wp-content/uploads/2021/06/PMS-and-menopause-March-22-update-final.pdf

Nicole, W. (2014). A Question for Women's Health: Chemicals in Feminine Hygiene Products and Personal Lubricants. *Environmental Health Perspectives, 122*(3), 70–75. https://doi.org/10.1289/ehp.122-a70

Nowakowski, S., Meers, J. M., & Heimbach, E. (2013). Sleep and Women's Health. *Sleep medicine research*, *4*(1), 1-22. https://doi.org/10.17241/smr.2013.4.1.1

Oates, J. (2017). The Effect of Yoga on Menstrual Disorders: A Systematic Review. *Journal of Alternative and Complementary Medicine, 23*(6), 407-417. https://doi.org/10.1089/acm.2016.0363

Peeters, C. (z.d.). *De enigmatische pathologie endometriose en de osteopathische benadering*. Osteopathie.be. https://osteopaatcolette.be/colette-in-vakpublicatie-about-osteopathy/?fbclid=IwAR1JX1oVuZMJH3D1CZZGcKJaWRBEYXmQkkeWpQpzZutdHMbzWLnGWSctzto

Pfaus, J. G., Quintana, G. R., Mac Cionnaith, C. E., & Parada, M. (2016). The whole versus the sum of some of the parts: toward resolving the apparent controversy of clitoral versus vaginal orgasms. *Socioaffective Neuroscience & Psychology*, *6*(1), 32578. https://doi.org/10.3402/snp.v6.32578

Pizzo, G., Giuliana, G., Milici, M. E., & Giangreco, R. (2000). Effect of dietary carbohydrates on the in vitro epithelial adhesion of Candida albicans, Candida tropicalis, and Candida krusei. *New Microbiol*, *23*(1), 63-71. https://pubmed.ncbi.nlm.nih.gov/10946407/

Pletzer, B., Harris, T., Scheuringer, A., & Hidalgo-Lopez, E. (2019). The cycling brain: menstrual cycle related fluctuations in hippocampal and fronto-striatal activation and connectivity during cognitive tasks. *Neuropsychopharmacology*, *44*(11), 1867-1875. https://doi.org/10.1038/s41386-019-0435-3

Ponce, M. M. (2017, 10 oktober). *Alles wat u moet weten over spotting* (Door Gyn&Co). Gyn&co. https://www.gynandco.be/nl/alles-wat-u-moet-weten-spotting/

Prasad, S., Tiwari, M., Pandey, A., Shrivastav, T. G., & Chaube, S. K. (2016). Impact of stress on oocyte quality and reproductive outcome. *Journal of Biomedical Science*, *23*(1), 36. https://doi.org/10.1186/s12929-016-0253-4

Raghunath, R. S., Venables, Z. C., & Millington, G. W. M. (2015). The menstrual cycle and the skin. *Clinical and Experimental Dermatology*, *40*(2), 111-115. https://doi.org/10.1111/ced.12588

Ranabir, S., & Reetu, K. (2011). Stress and hormones. *Indian Journal of Endocrinology and Metabolism*, *15*(1), 18. https://doi.org/10.4103/2230-8210.77573

Rani, K., Tiwari, S., Kumar, S., Singh, U., Prakash, J., & Srivastava, N. (2016). The Effect of Yoga Nidra on Psychological Problems of Women with Menstrual Disorders: a Randomized Clinical Trial. *Journal of Caring Sciences*, *5*(1), 1-9. https://doi.org/10.15171/jcs.2016.001

Reimers, L., Büchel, C., & Diekhof, E. K. (2014). How to be patient. The ability to wait for a reward depends on the phase of the menstrual cycle and feedback-related activity. *Frontiers in Neuroscience*, *8*, 401. https://doi.org/10.3389/fnins.2014.00401

Rizzoli, R., Biver, E., & Brennan-Speranza, T. C. (2021). Nutritional intake and bone health. *The Lancet Diabetes & Endocrinology*, *9*(9), 606-621. https://doi.org/10.1016/s2213-8587(21)00119-4

Rossi, M. (2021). Love Your Gut: *Supercharge Your Digestive Health and Transform Your Well-Being from the Inside Out*. The Experiment.

Santoro, N. (2016). Perimenopause: From Research to Practice. *Journal of Womens Health*, *25*(4), 332-339. https://doi.org/10.1089/jwh.2015.5556

Schoep, M. E., Adang, E. M. M., Maas, J. W., De Bie, B., Aarts, J. W., & Nieboer, T. E. (2019a). Productivity loss due to menstruation-related symptoms: a nationwide cross-sectional survey among 32 748 women. *BMJ Open*, *9*(6), e026186. https://doi.org/10.1136/bmjopen-2018-026186

Shah, A. (2021). I'm So Effing Tired: *A proven plan to beat burnout, boost your energy and reclaim your life*. Harvest Publications.

Shechter, A., Varin, F., & Boivin, D. B. (2010). Circadian Variation of Sleep During the Follicular and Luteal Phases of the Menstrual Cycle. *Sleep*, *33*(5), 647-656. https://doi.org/10.1093/sleep/33.5.647

Stichting PMDD Nederland. (z.d.). *Wat is PMDD?* PMDD Nederland. https://www.pmddnederland.nl/wat-is-pmdd?gclid=Cj0KCQiAj4ecBhD3ARIsAM4Q_jGTwKfZQPknNjmdA2D_vmRQ2xsWMU0h6TdQkKlmvrbtvmvLpVID6xYaArQREALw_wcB

8Szczuko, M., Kikut, J., Szczuko, U., Szydłowska, I., Nawrocka-Rutkowska, J., Ziętek, M., Verbanac, D., & Saso, L. (2021). Nutrition Strategy and Life Style in Polycystic Ovary Syndrome—Narrative Review. *Nutrients*, *13*(7), 2452. https://doi.org/10.3390/nu13072452

Team Isala. (2022, 4 juli). *Isala newsflash: verschillende factoren hebben een impact op je vaginale microbioom*. Isala. https://isala.be/isala-newsflash-verschillende-factoren-hebben-een-impact-op-je-vaginale-microbioom/

van de Wiel, H. B. M. (2011, 1 januari). *Premenstrueel syndroom (PMS)* (Door Federatie Medisch Specialisten). Richtlijnendatabase.nl. https://richtlijnendatabase.nl/richtlijn/premenstrueel_syndroom/pms_-_algemene_inleiding.html

Van Hoeven, F. (2021, 21 november). *Van depressie tot hartfalen: waarom er meer medische aandacht voor vrouwen nodig is*. Eva Jinek. https://www.evajinek.nl/onderwerpen/artikel/5268288/vrouwen-geneeskunde-medicatie-aandoening-hart-hormonen-cyclus

Vargas, S. L., Patrick, C. C., Ayers, G. D., & Hughes, W. T. (1993). Modulating effect of dietary carbohydrate supplementation on Candida albicans colonization and invasion in a neutropenic mouse model. *Infection and Immunity*, *61*(2), 619-626. https://doi.org/10.1128/iai.61.2.619-626.1993

Volpi, E., Nazemi, R., & Fujita, S. (2004). Muscle tissue changes with aging. *Current Opinion in Clinical Nutrition and Metabolic Care*, *7*(4), 405-410. https://doi.org/10.1097/01.mco.0000134362.76653.b2

Watson, S. (August 20, 2018). *All About the Luteal Phase of the Menstrual Cycle*. Healthline. https://www.healthline.com/health/womens-health/luteal-phase#short-luteal-phase

Wear White Again. (September 24, 2018). *Heavy Periods market research - results summary*. Google Docs. https://drive.google.com/file/d/1uVgpuHita5teXyTGYQguDIOJRLBB9b0O/view

Wong, C. (June 25, 2022). *What Hormone Imbalance Tests Reveal About Women's Health*. Verywell Health. https://www.verywellhealth.com/hormone-blood-test-for-women-89722

Xenou, M., & Gourounti, K. (2021). Dietary Patterns and Polycystic Ovary Syndrome: a Systematic Review. *Mædica*, *16*(3). https://doi.org/10.26574/maedica.2020.16.3.516

Yang, Z., & Schank, J. C. (2006). Women do not synchronize their menstrual cycles. *Human Nature*, *17*(4), 433-447. https://doi.org/10.1007/s12110-006-1005-z

Ziekenhuis.nl, & Middelburg, J. (2017, 27 november). *Ethinylestradiol - Medicijnen*. Ziekenhuis.nl. https://www.ziekenhuis.nl/medicijnen/e/ethinylestradiol/item29475

Colophon

www.lannoo.com

Register on our website and we will regularly send you a newsletter with information about new books and interesting, exclusive offers.

Editorial: Sofie Vanherpe

Illustrations: Zinzi Moons

Design: Tina De Souter

We have respected the copyright attributions of the quotes found, but were unable to identify some of the references. If you are the owner of any of the quotes in this book, please contact our editorial team.

If you have any comments or questions, you can contact our editorial team at redactielifestyle@lannoo.com.

D/2024/45/577 - NUR 860 / 450

ISBN: 978 90 209 5598 9